RETIRED NURSE

ADULT
COLORING BOOK

Enjoying this book?

Please leave a review because we would love to know your thoughts, feedback, and opinions to create better paper products for you!

Thank you so much for your support.

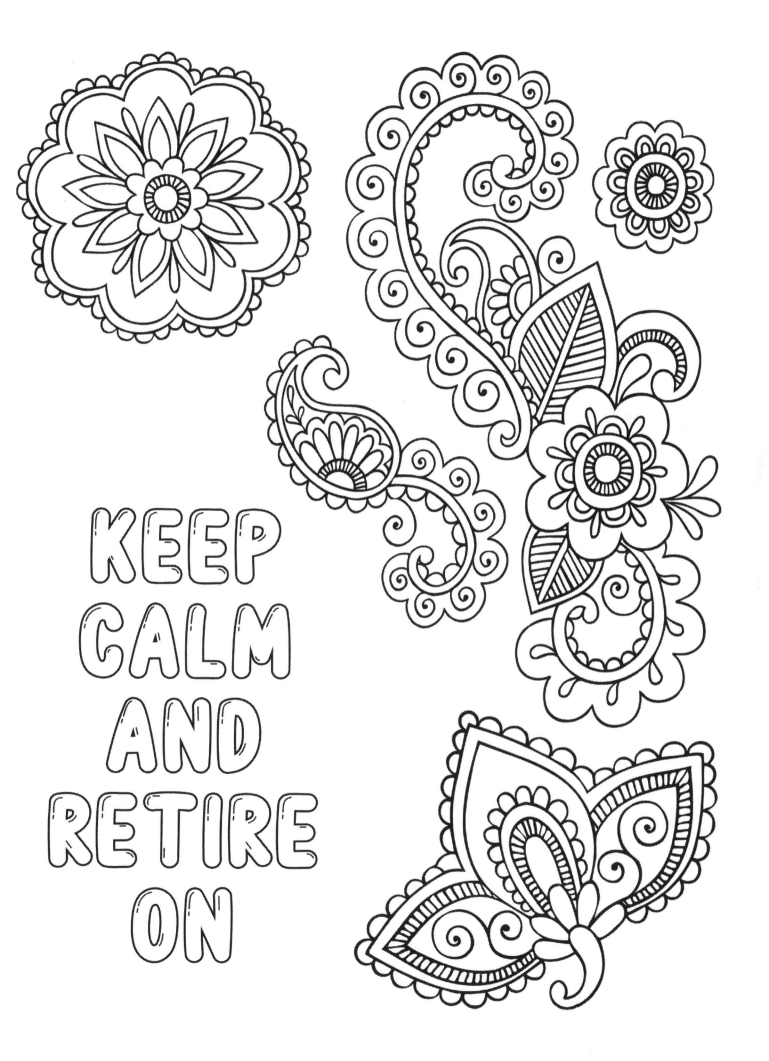

KEEP CALM AND RETIRE ON

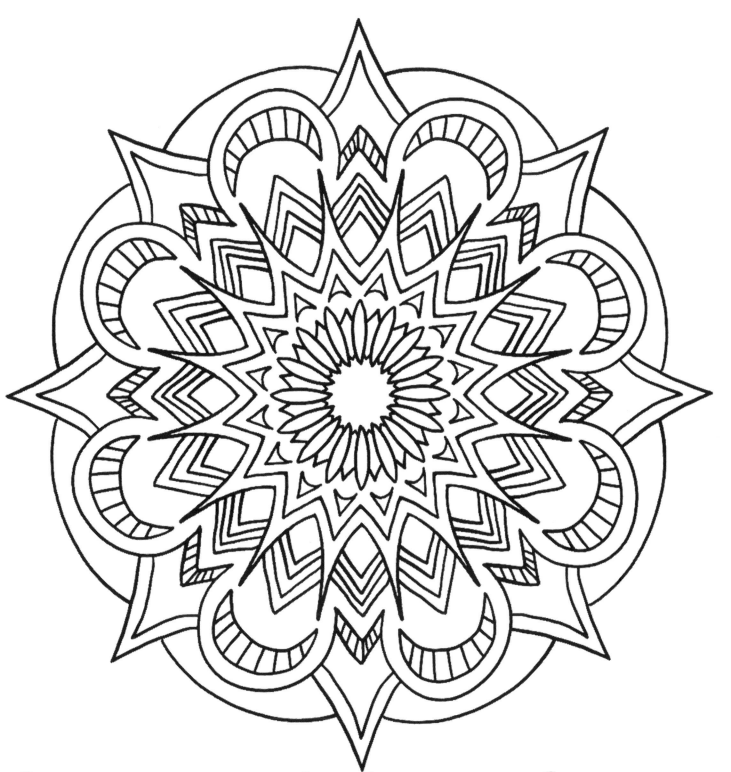

Laughter is the best medicine...
except for
treating diarrhea...

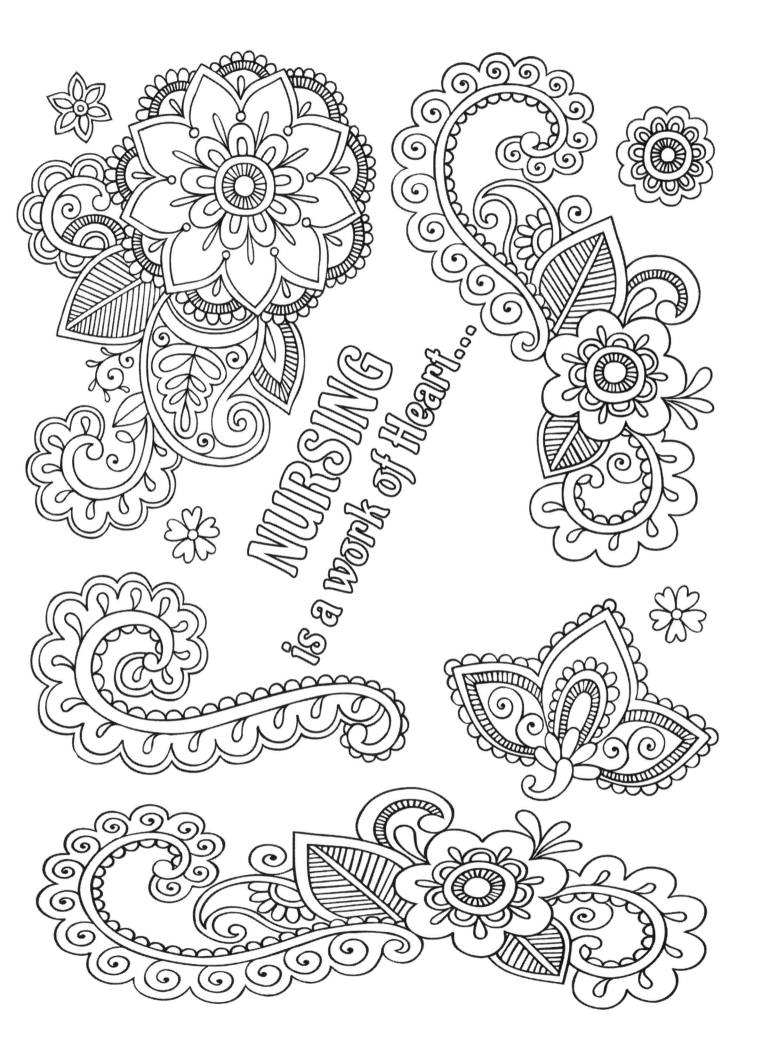

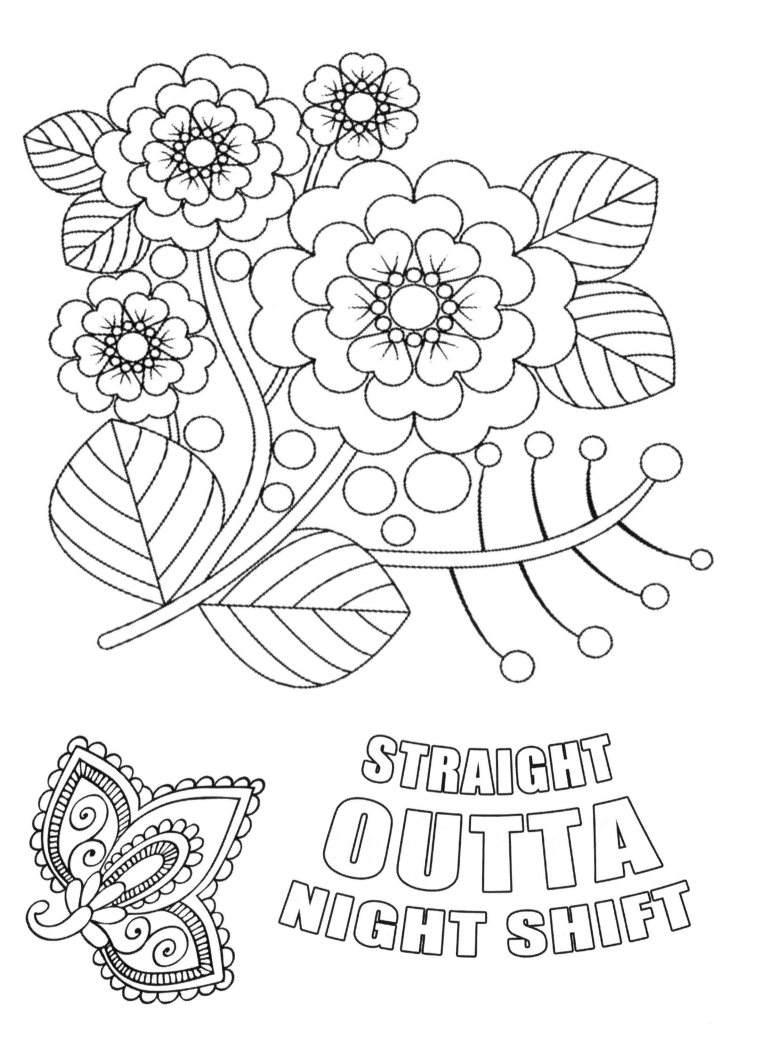

STRAIGHT OUTTA NIGHT SHIFT

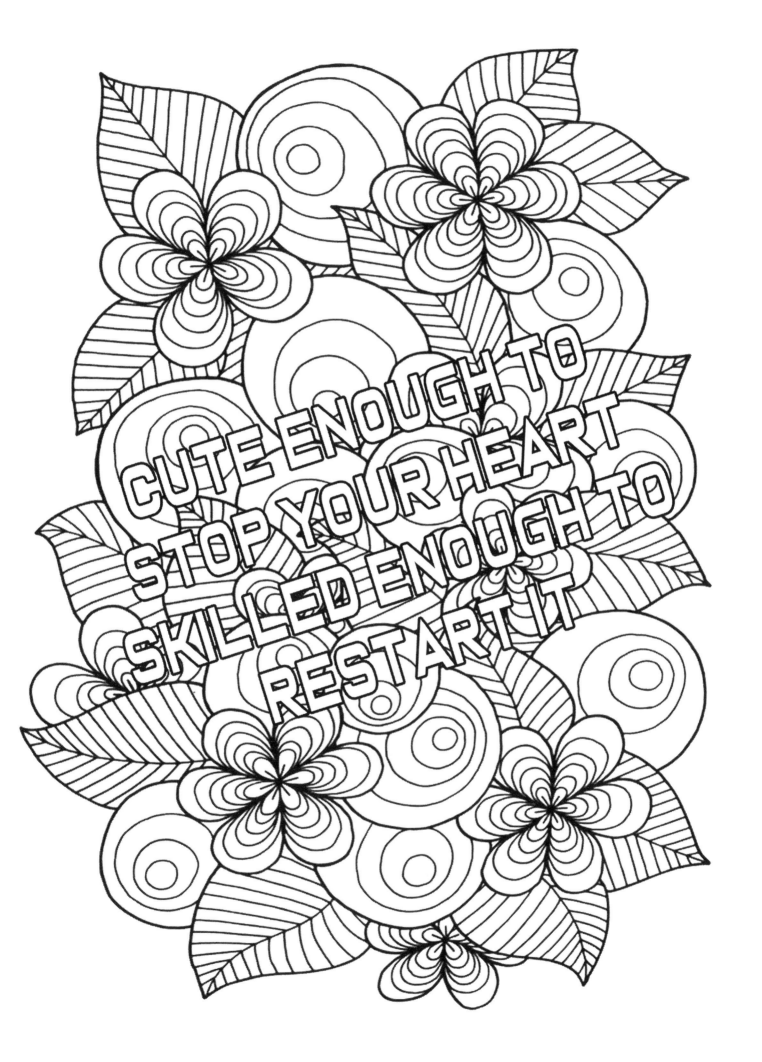

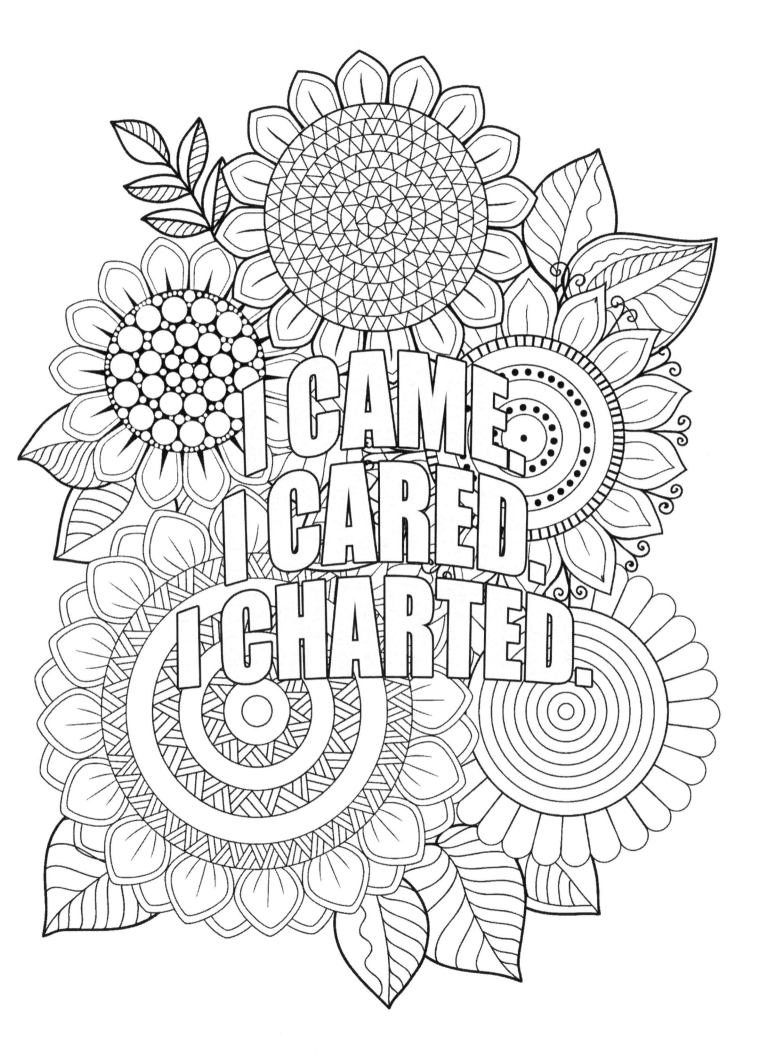

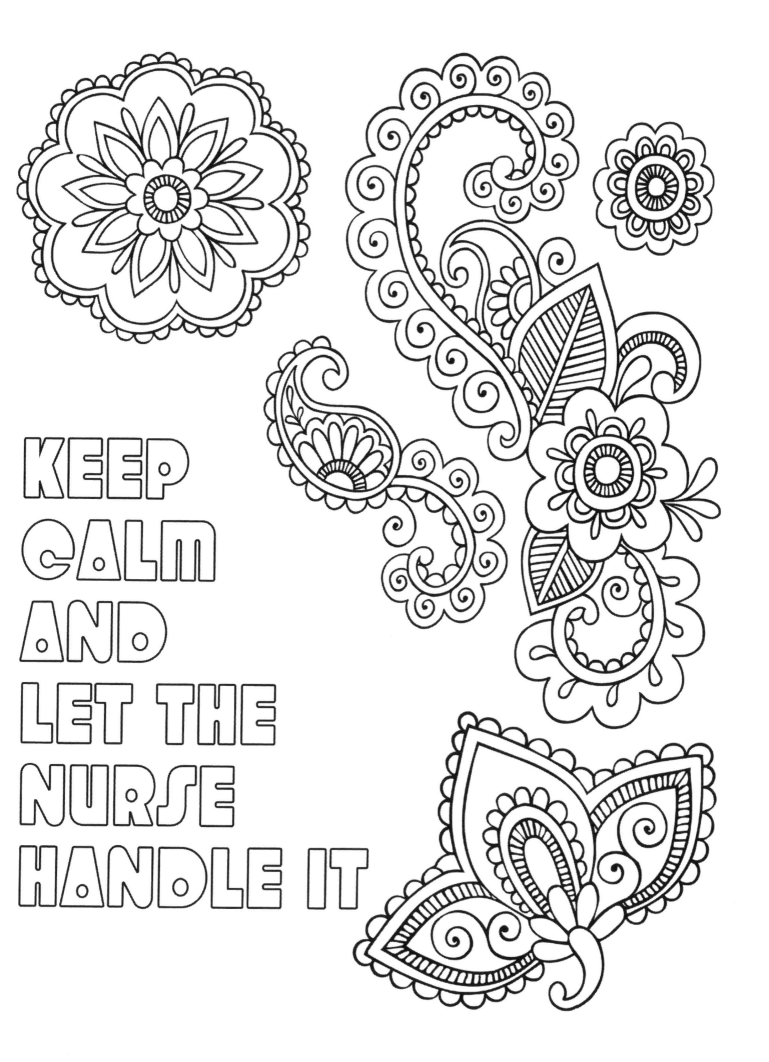

KEEP CALM AND LET THE NURSE HANDLE IT

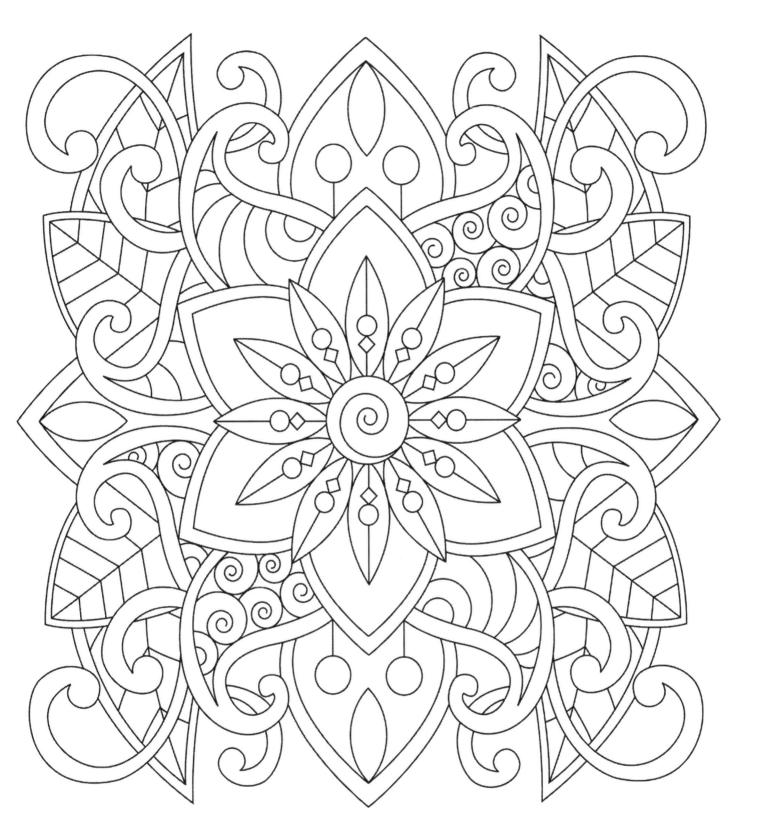

"No, RN does not stand for Refreshments and Narcotics"

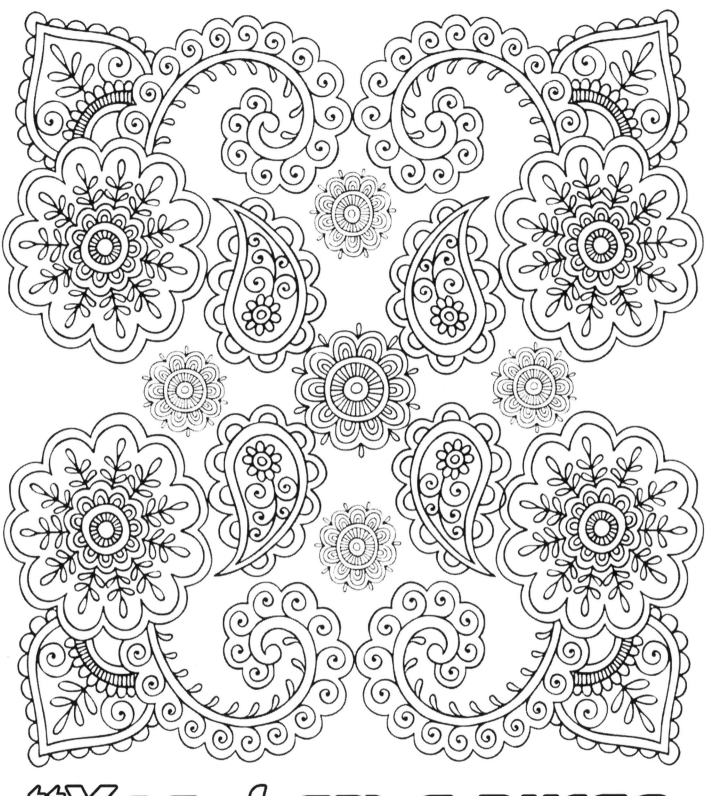

"Yes, I am a nurse. No, I don't want to look at it."

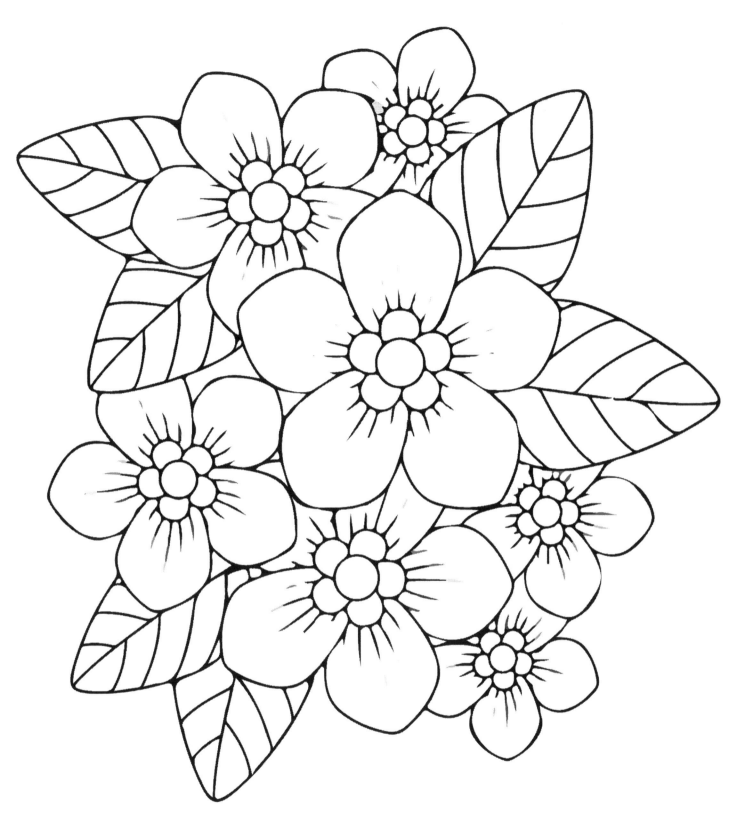

YOU CAN'T CURE STUPID, BUT YOU CAN SEDATE IT.

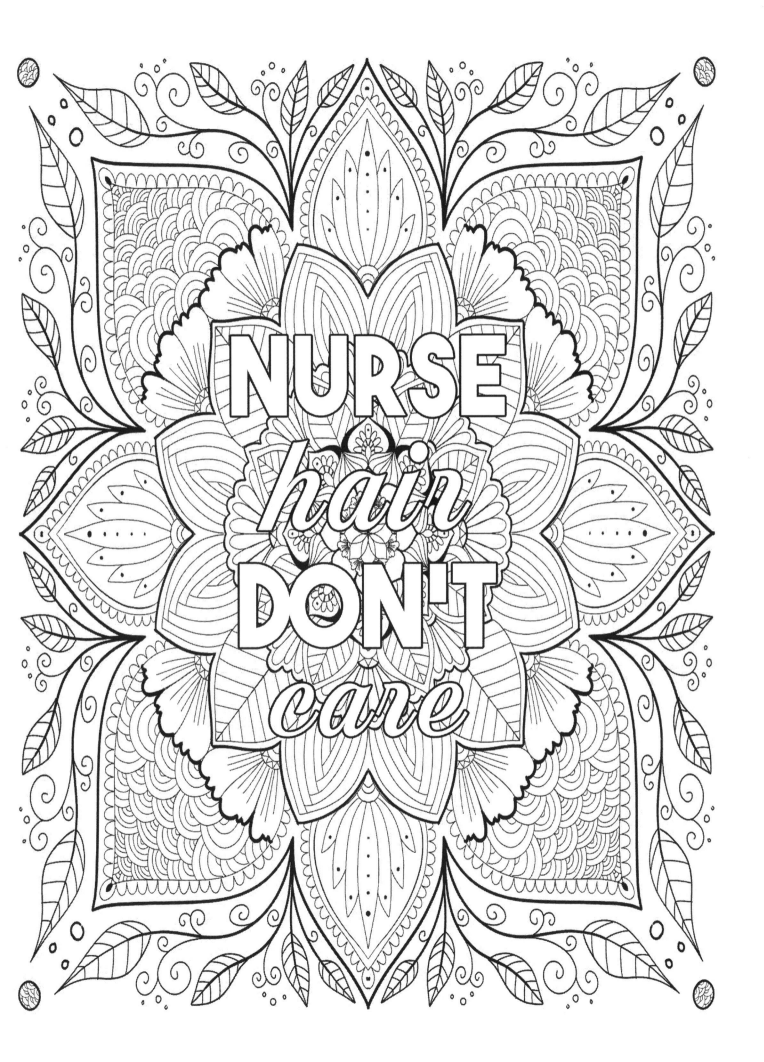

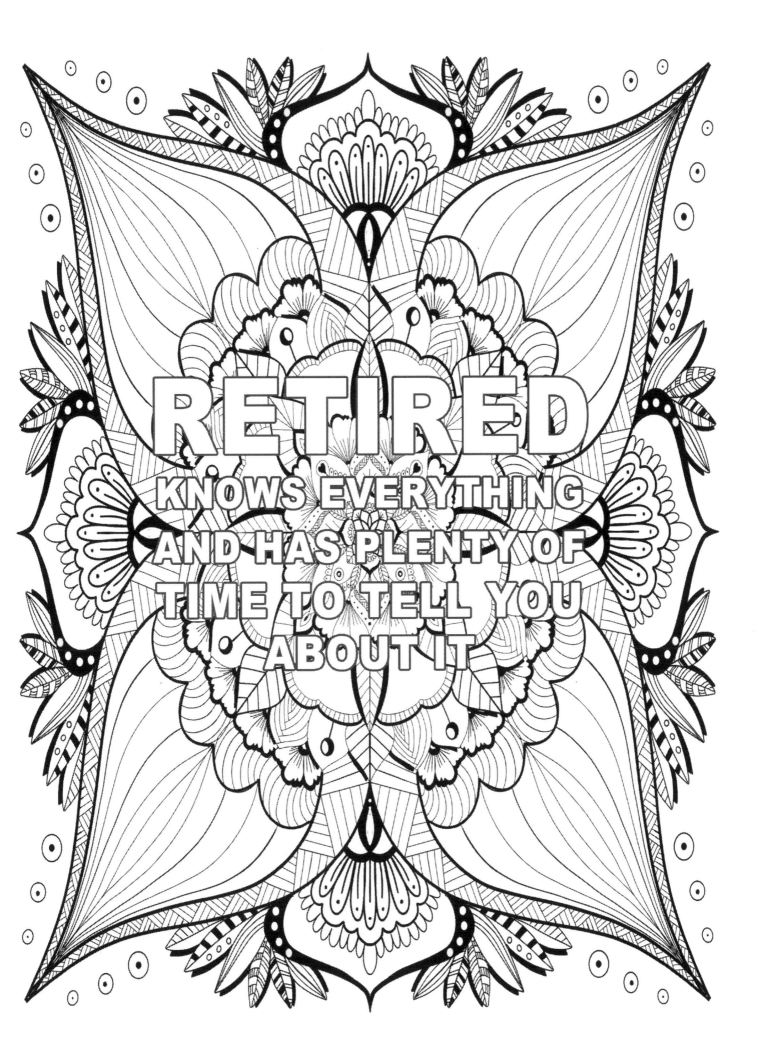

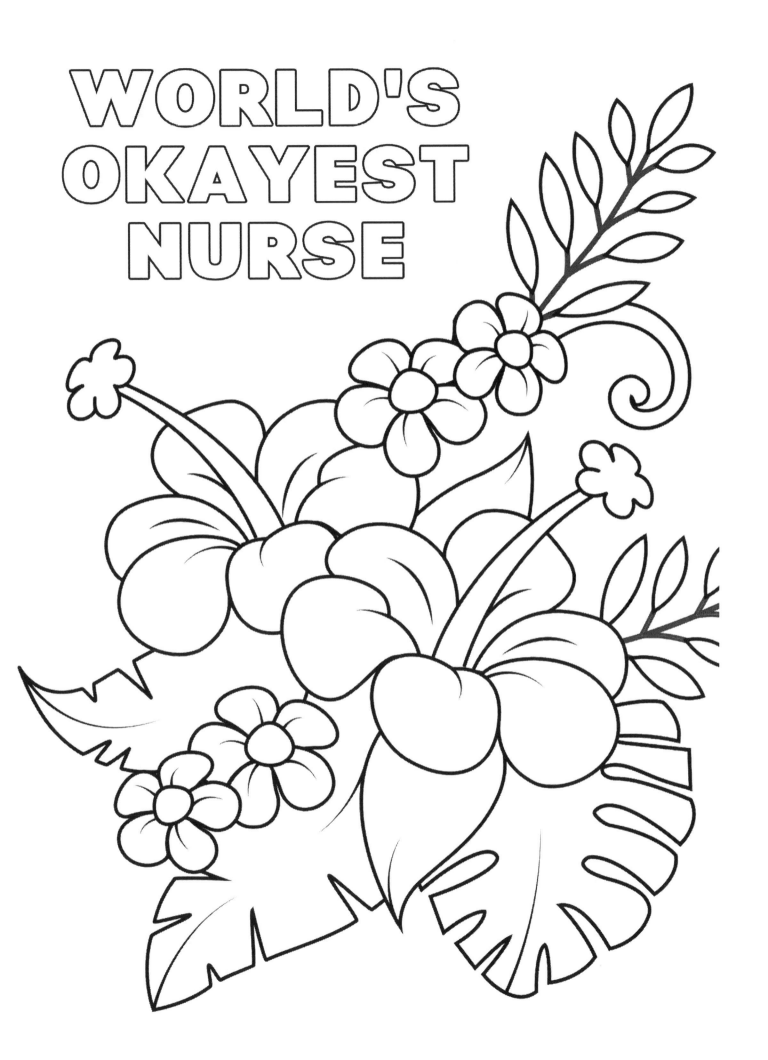

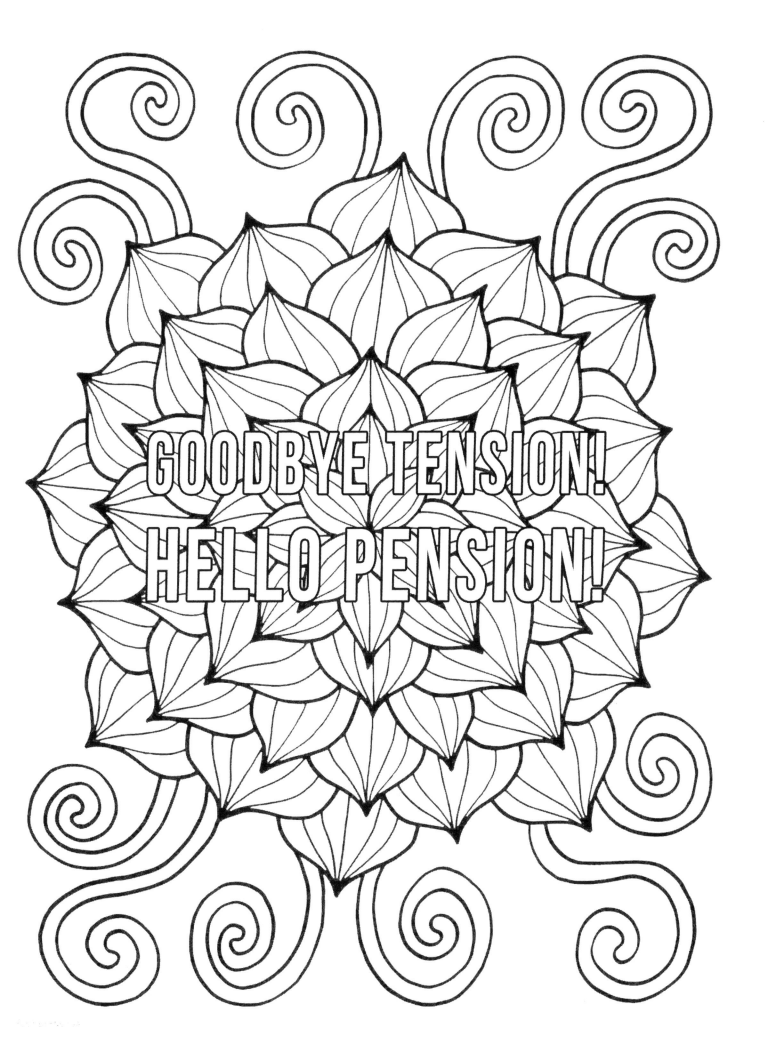

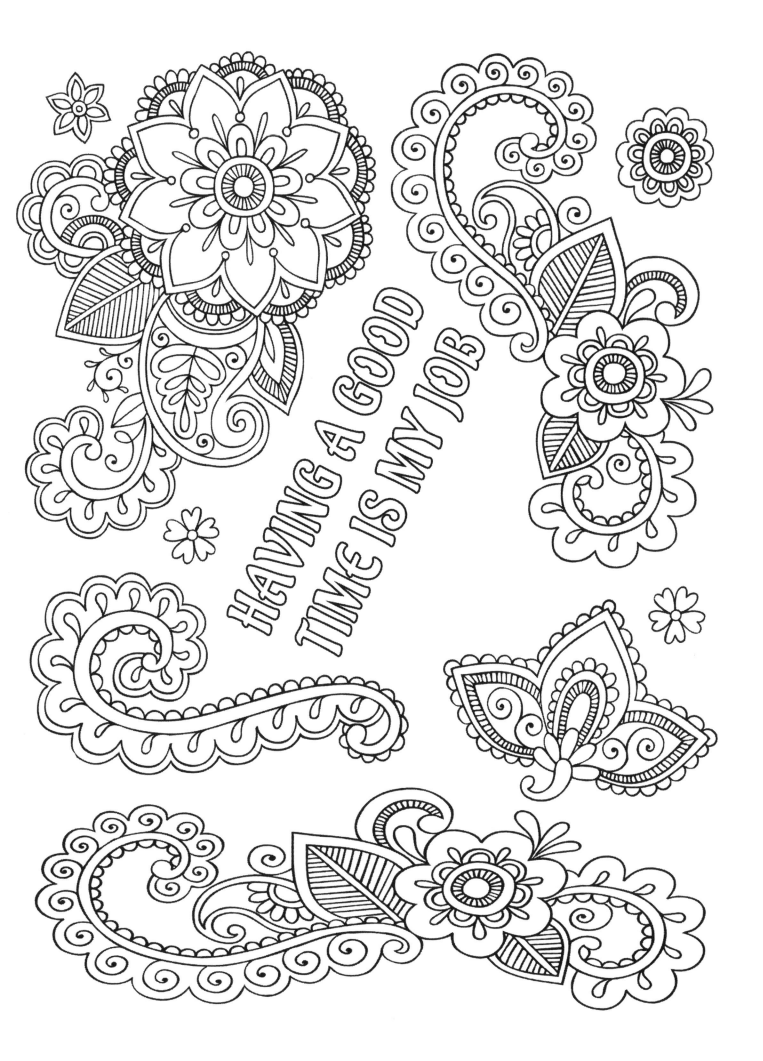

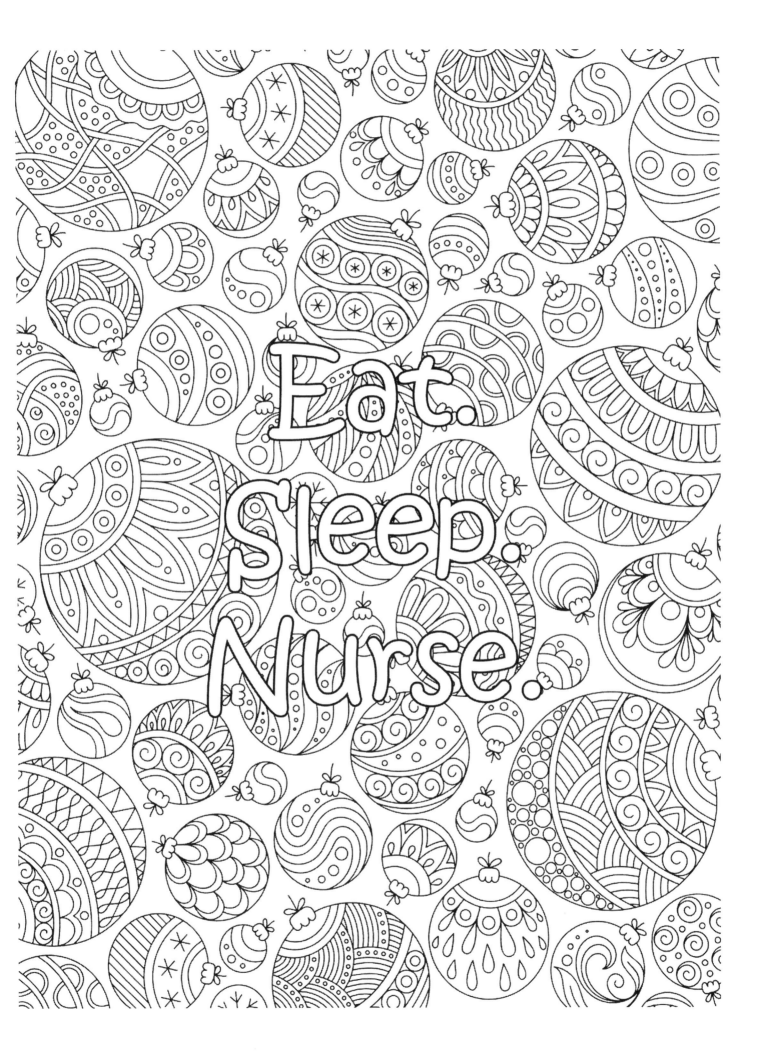

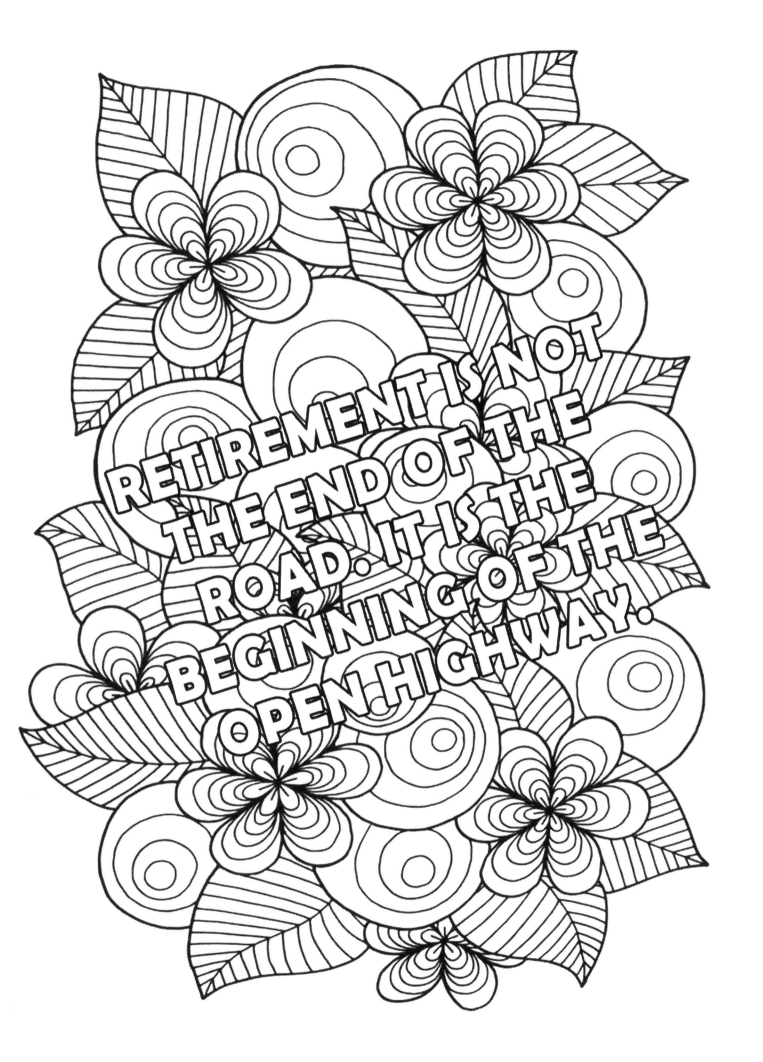

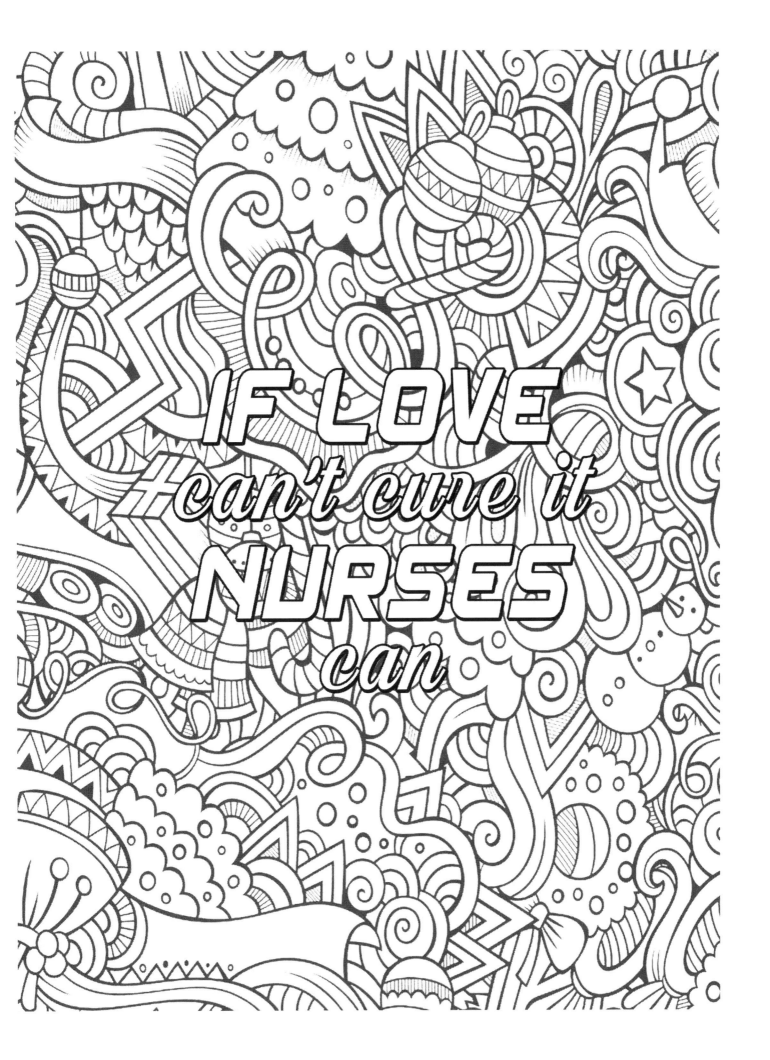

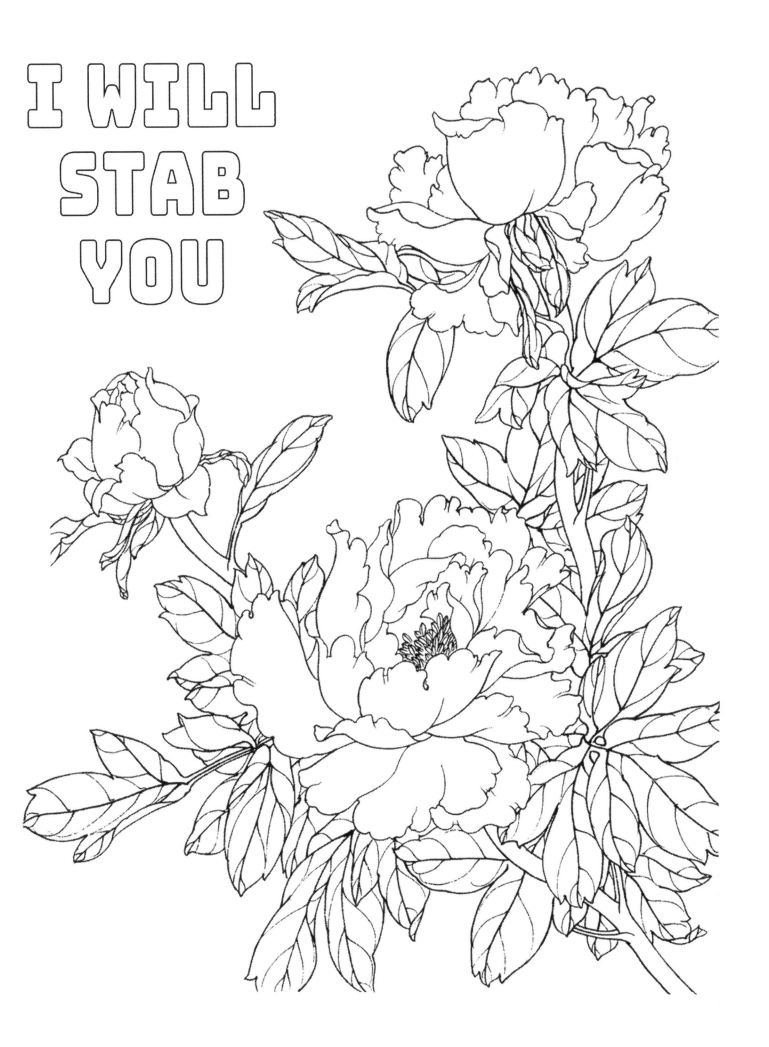

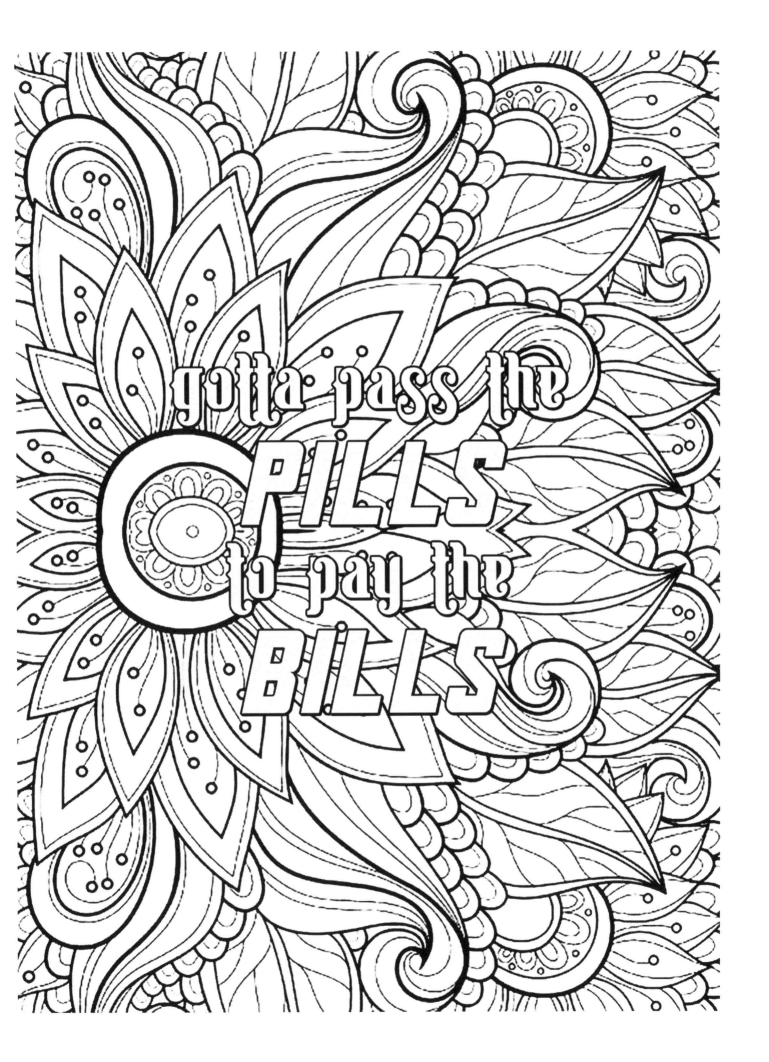

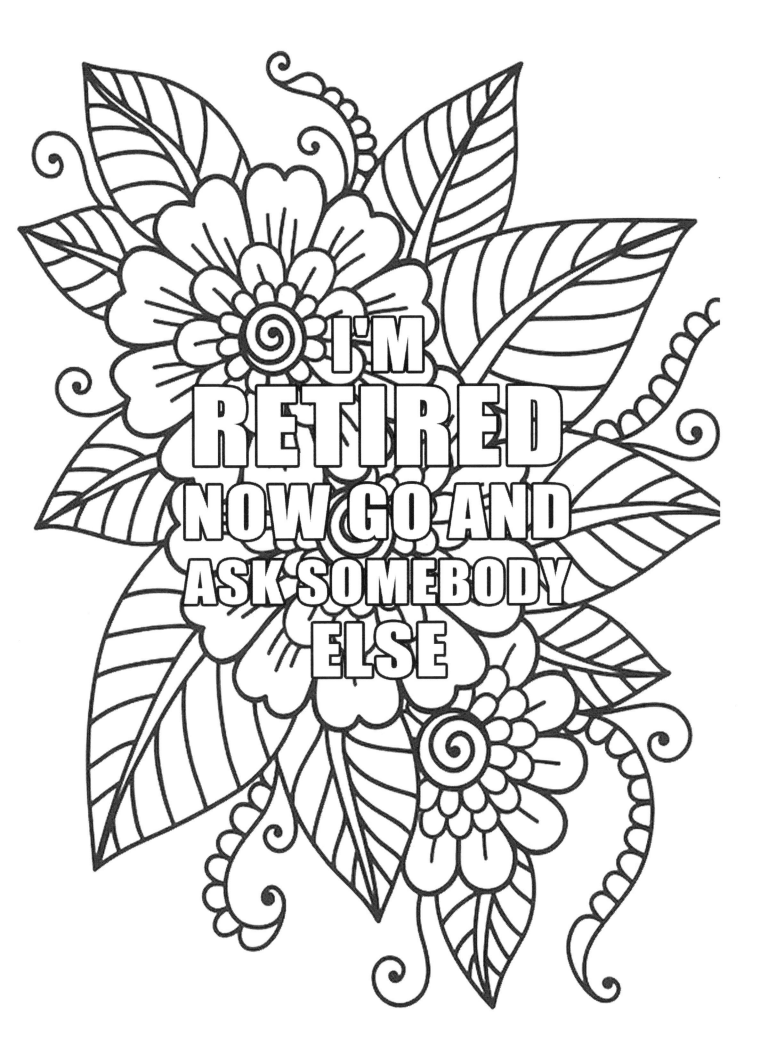

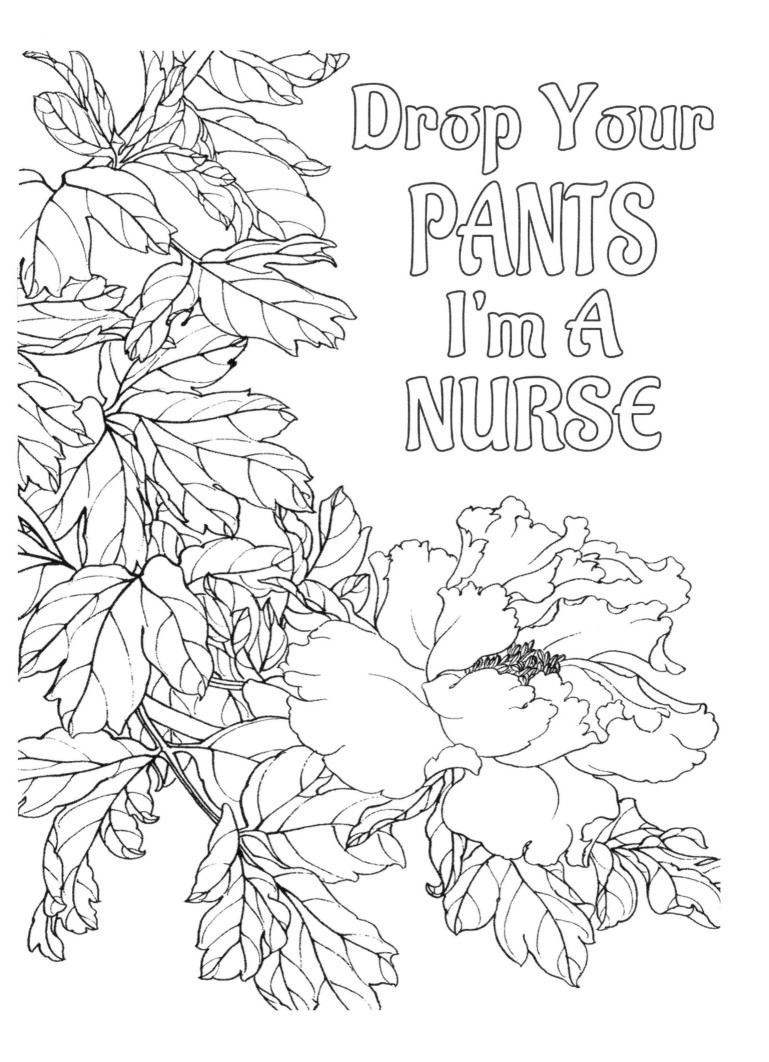

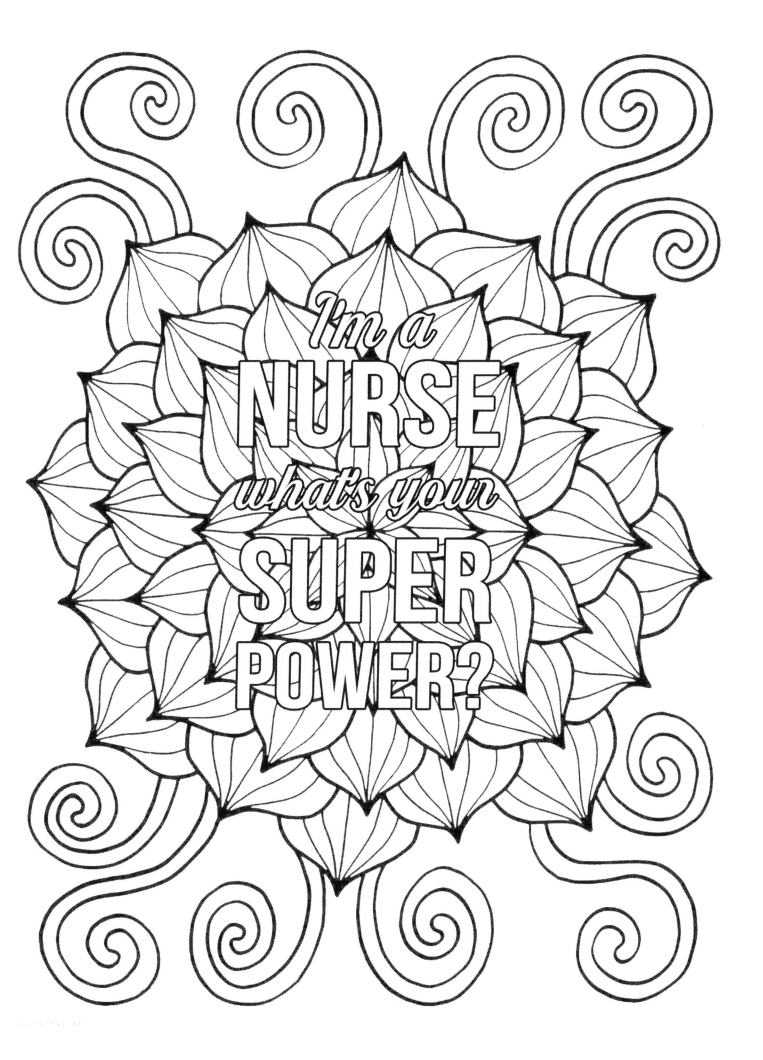

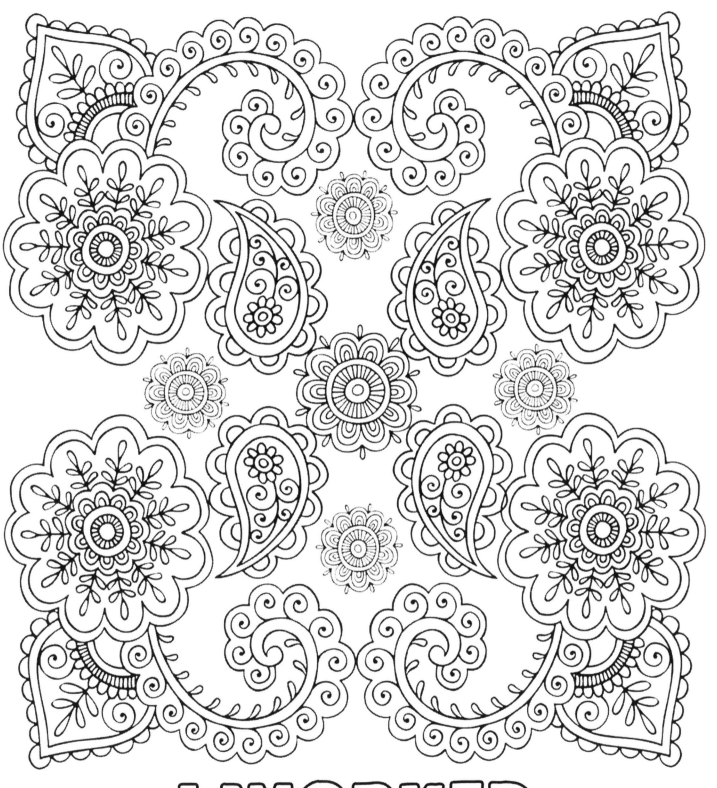

I WORKED
MY WHOLE LIFE
FOR THIS BOOK

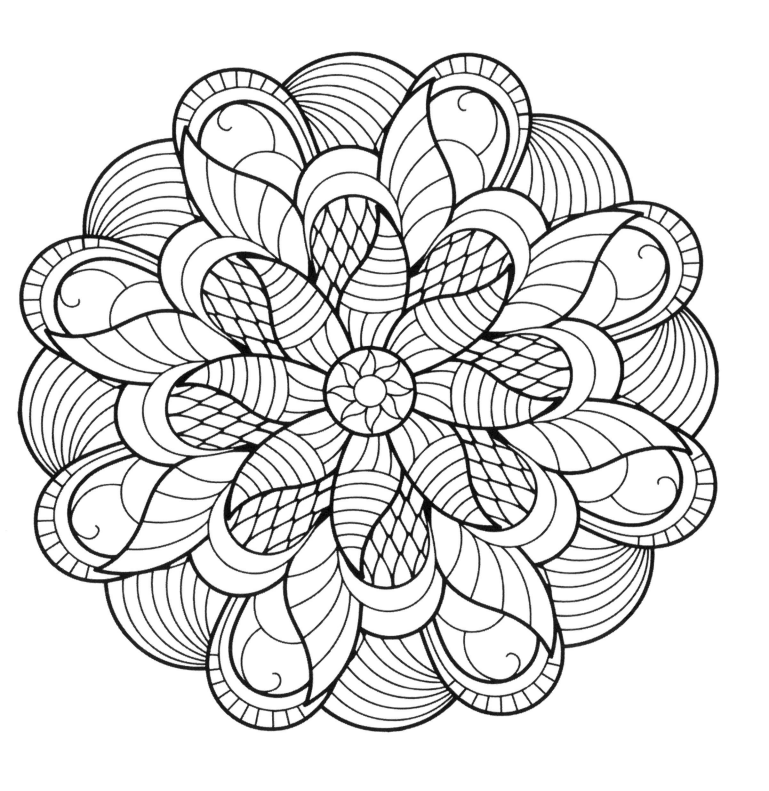

NURSES, LET'S CELEBRATE
OUR ABILITY TO HOLD
IN OUR PEE FOR 10 HOURS

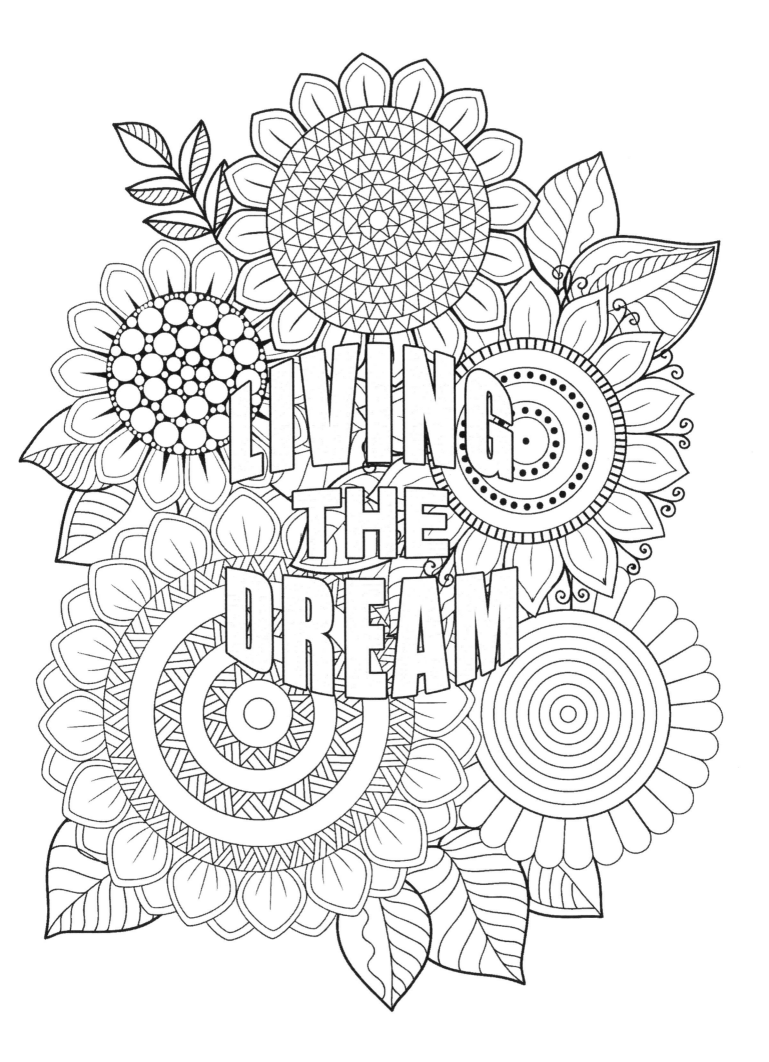

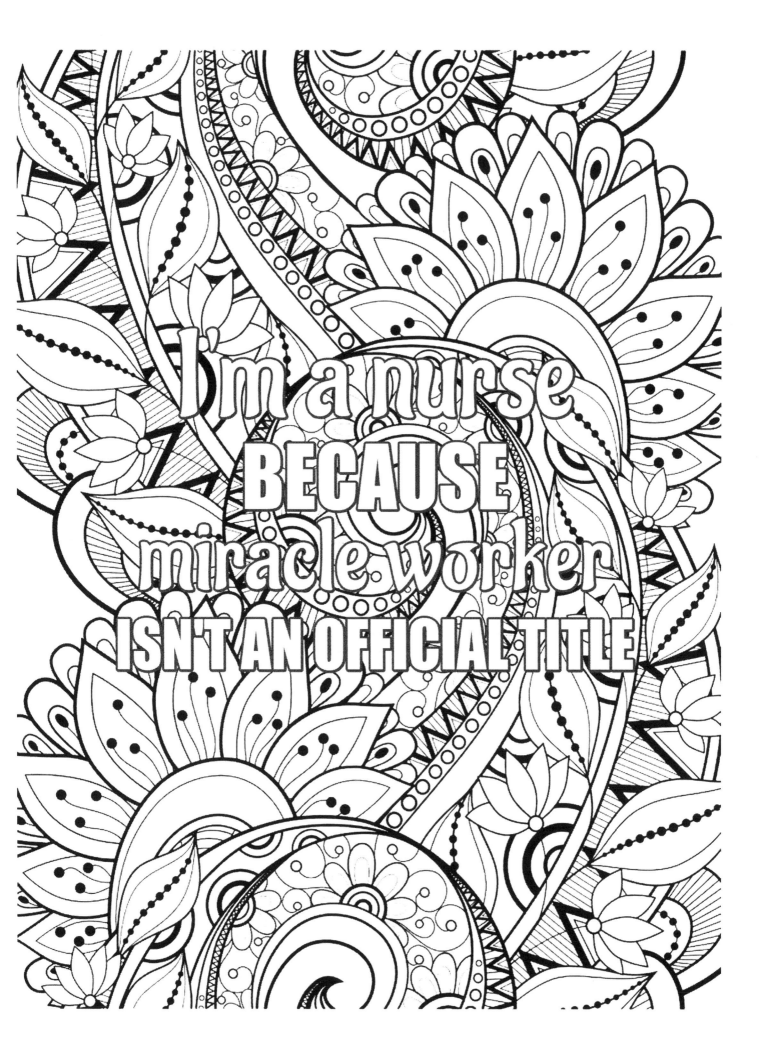

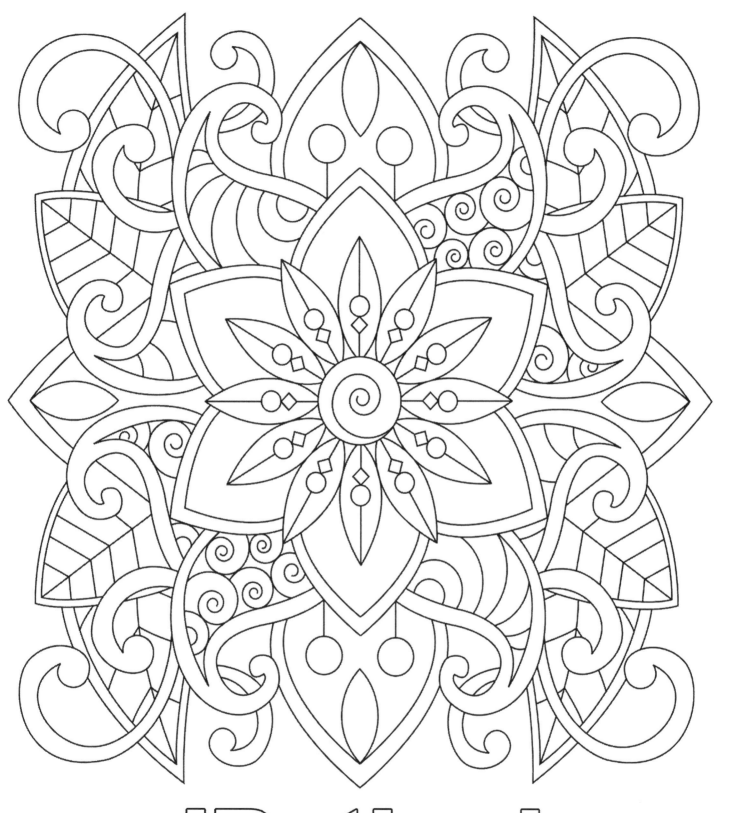

iRetired
There's a nap for that

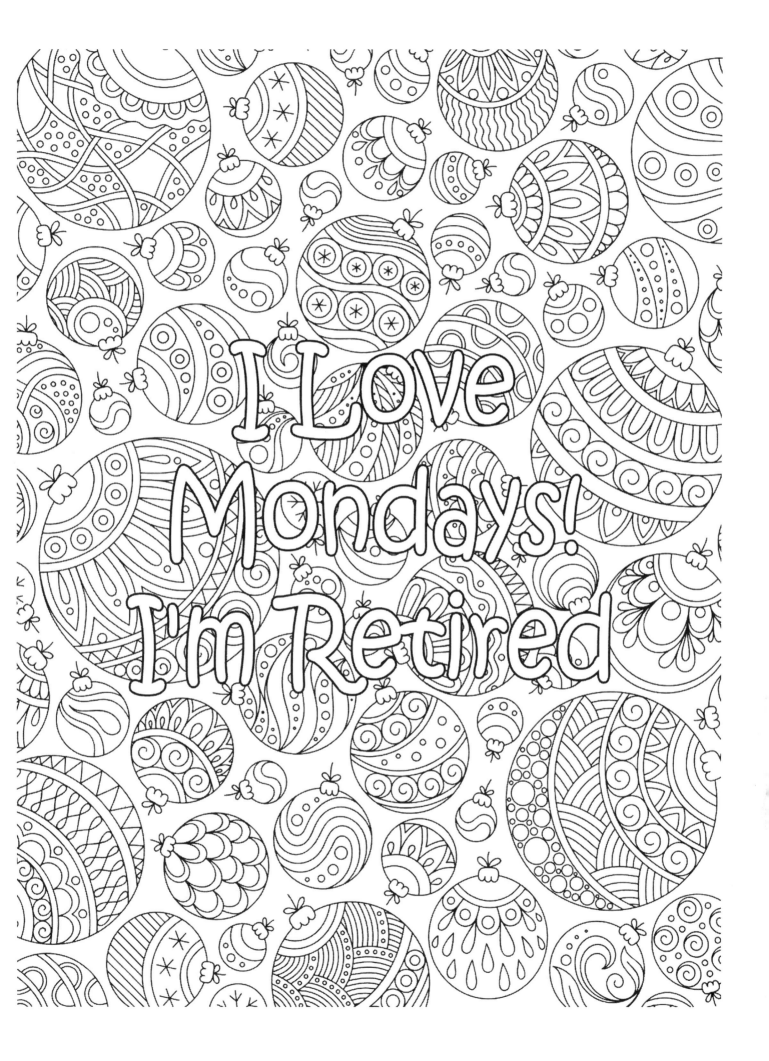

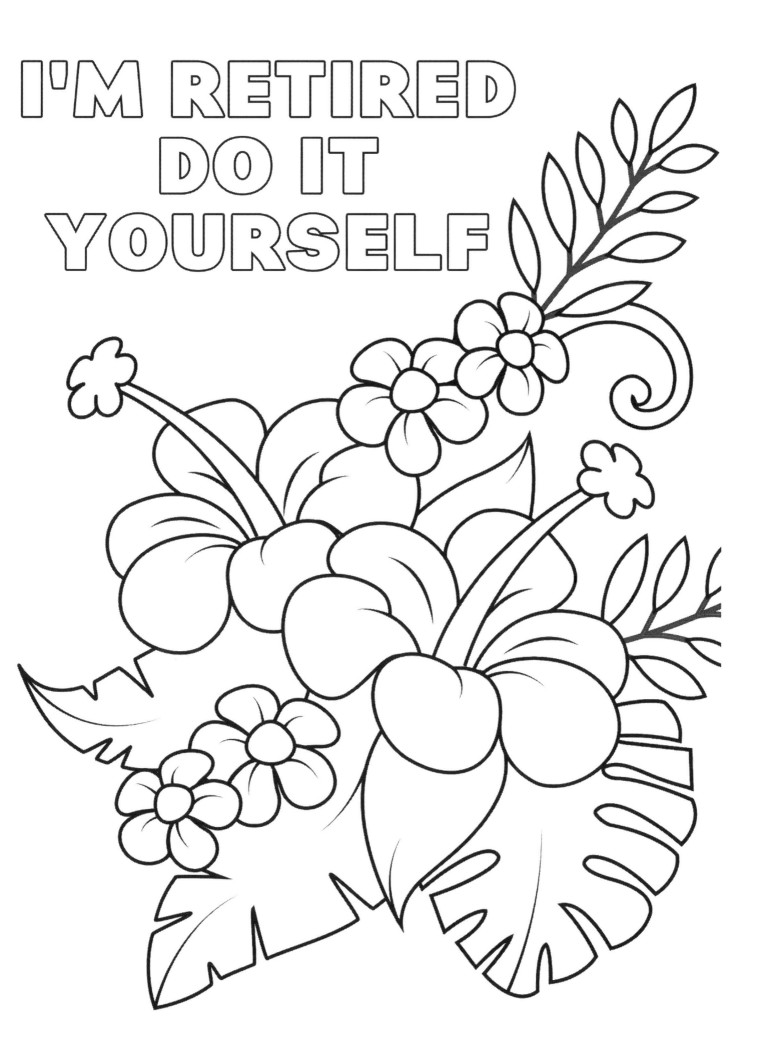

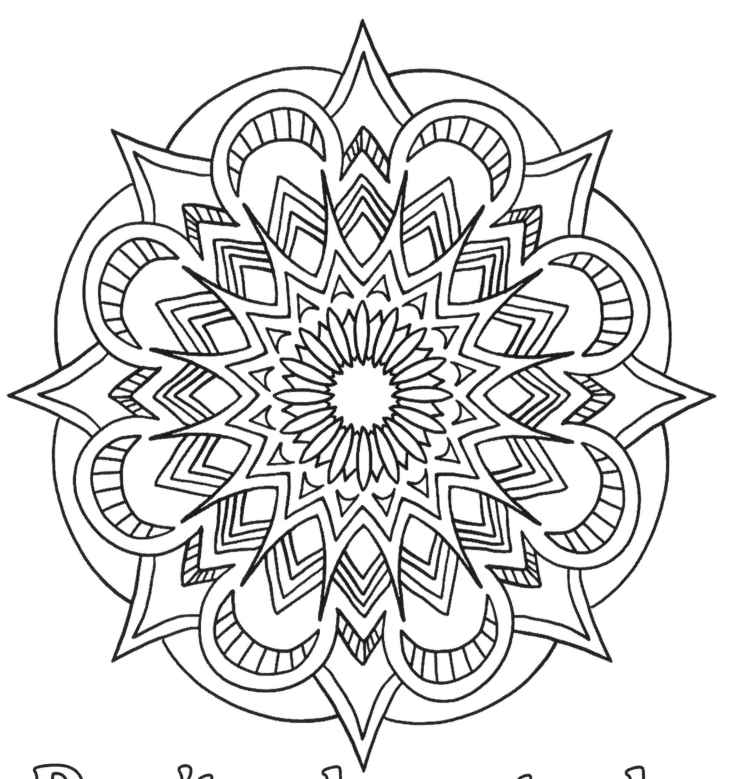

Don't ask me to do
one damn thing.
I'm Retired

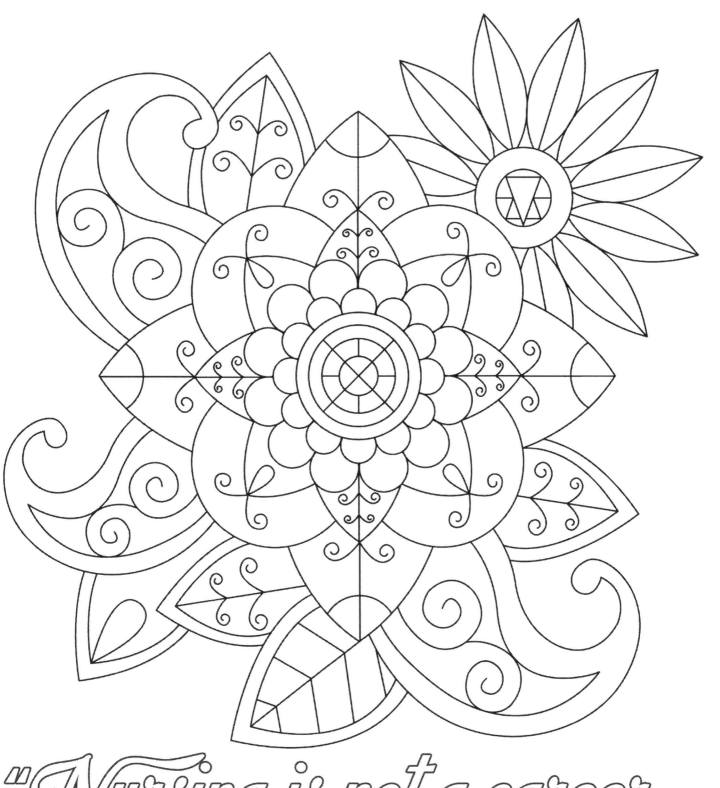

"Nursing is not a career...
its a post-apocalyptic
survival skill"

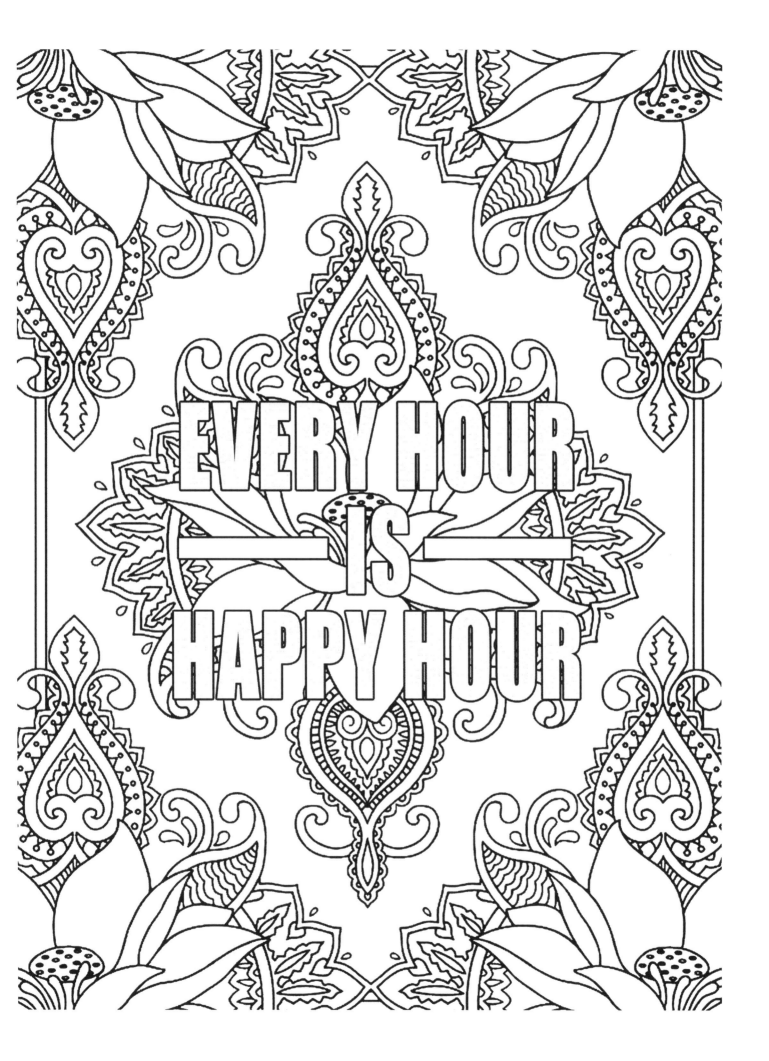

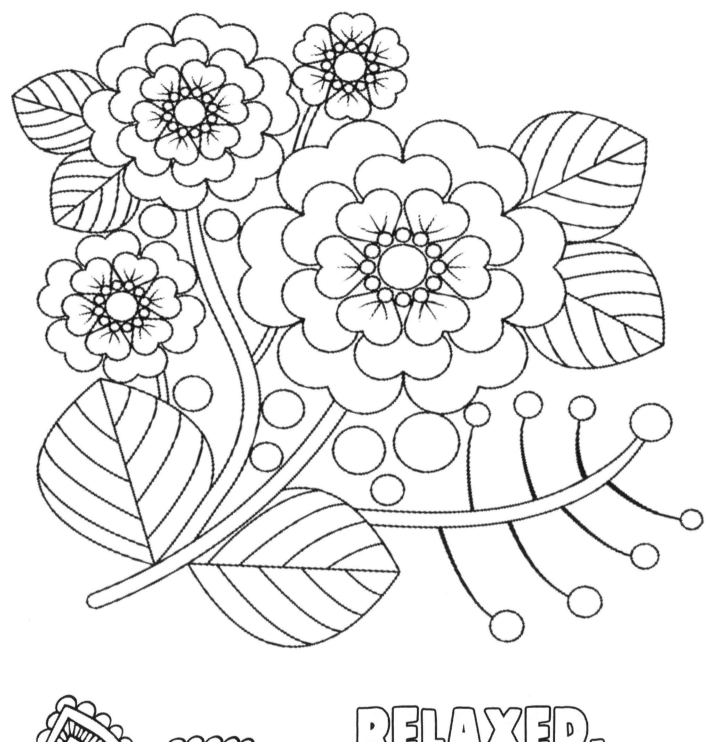

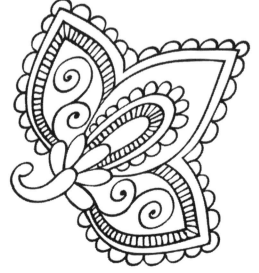

RELAXED.
RENEWED.
Retired!

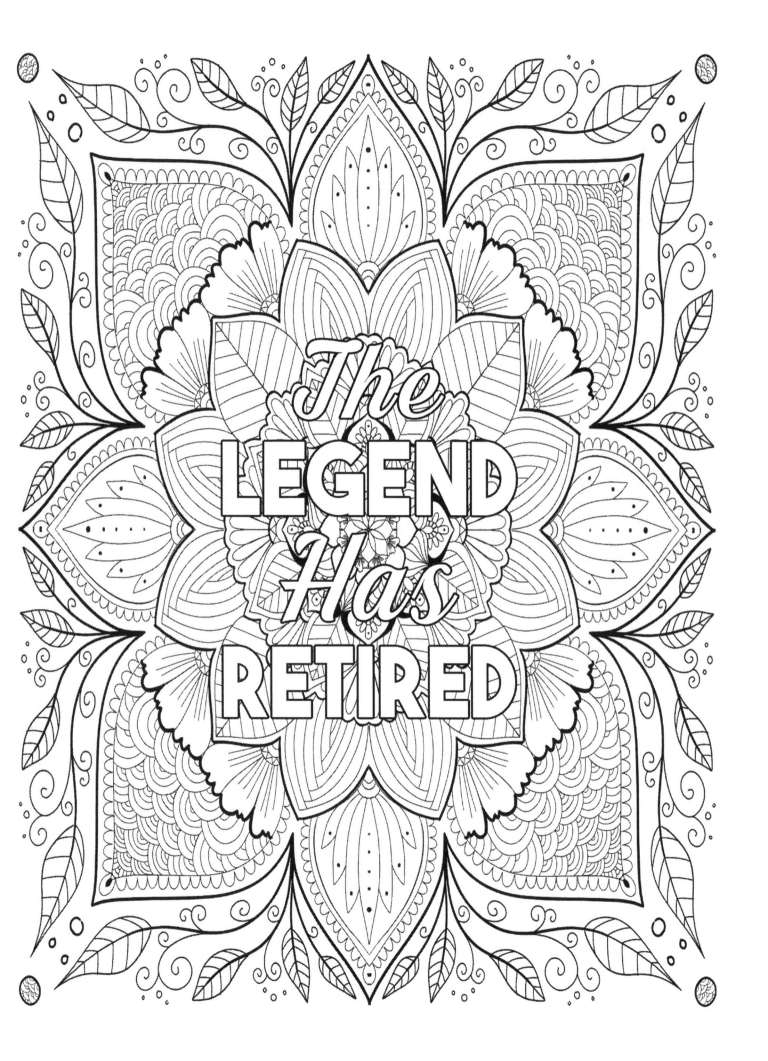

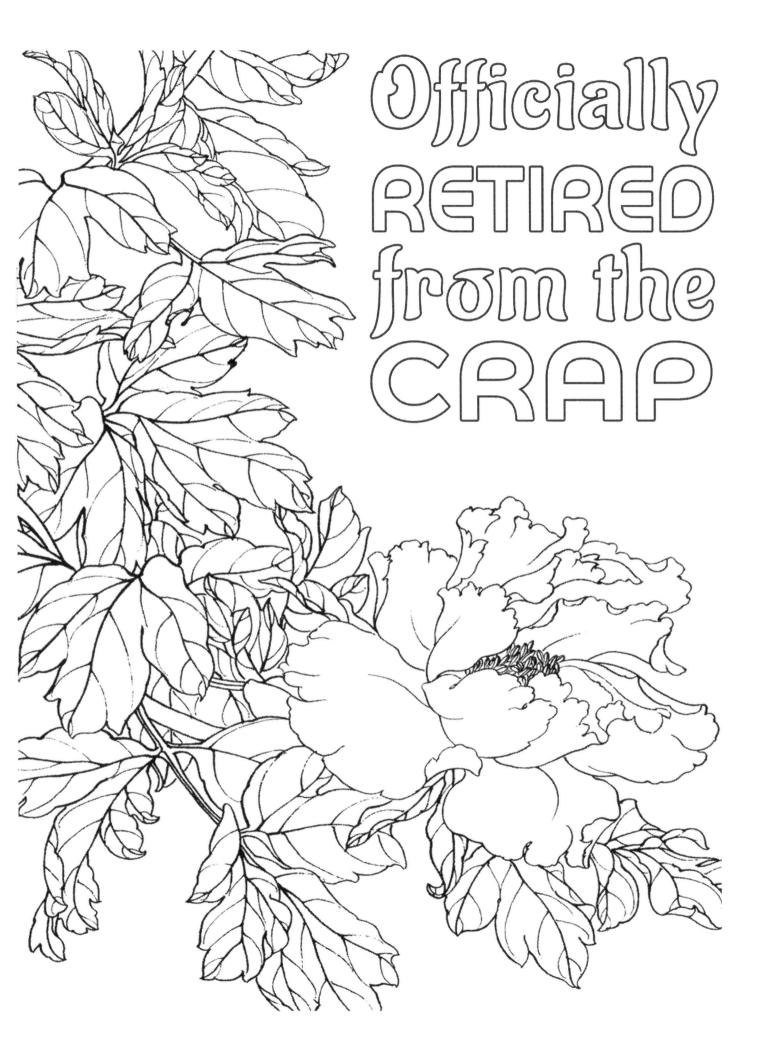

WISHING YOU A SPEEDY RECOVERY FROM YOUR IMAGINARY ILLNESS.

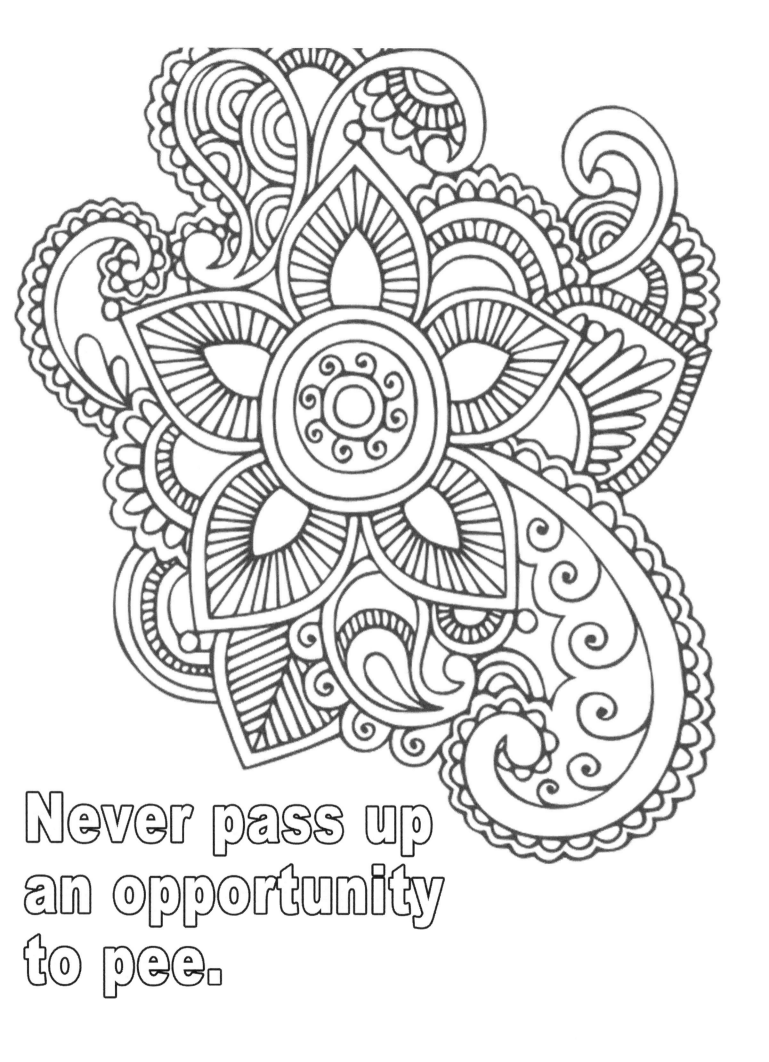

Never pass up
an opportunity
to pee.

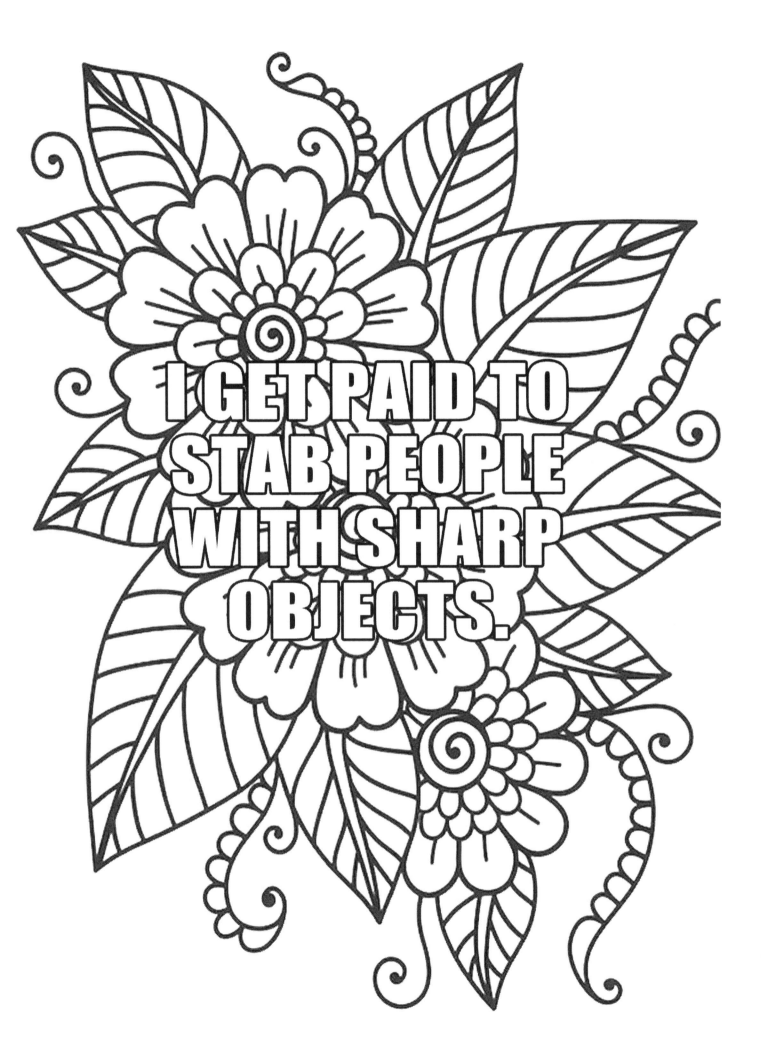

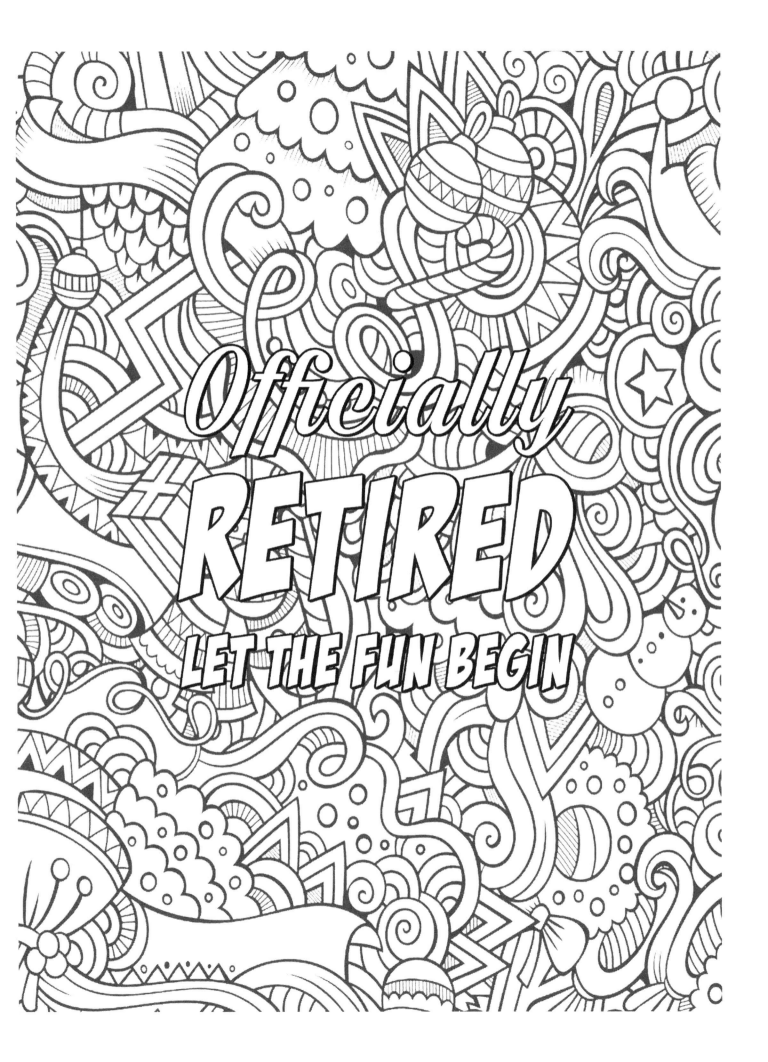

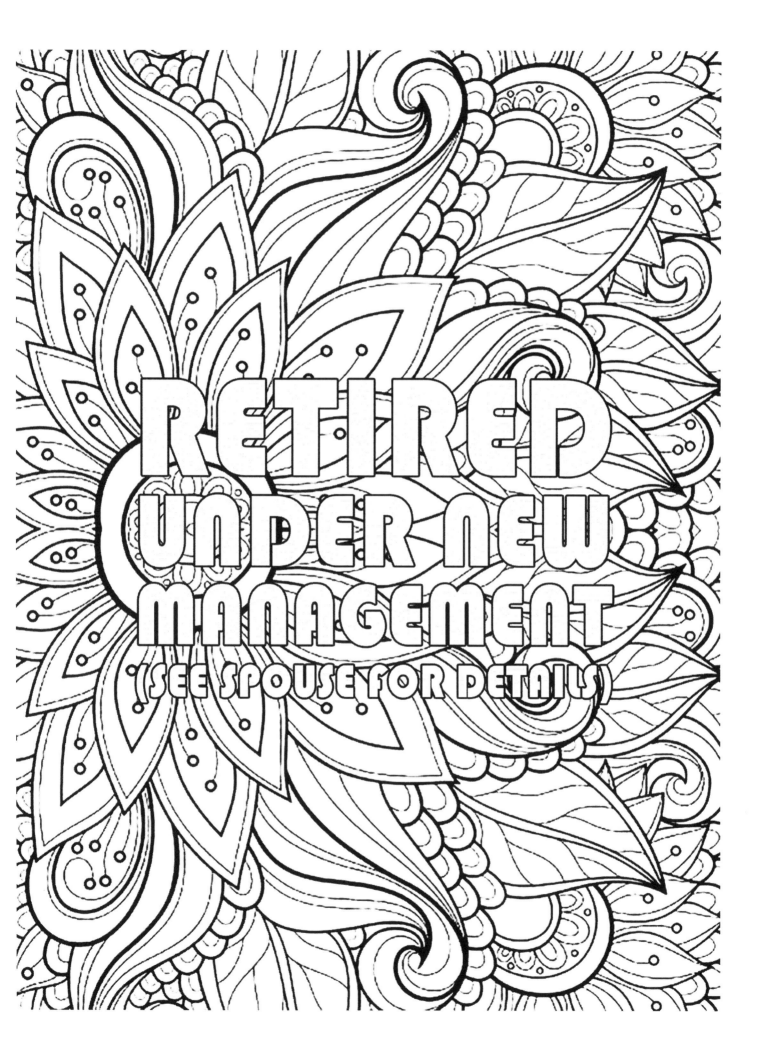

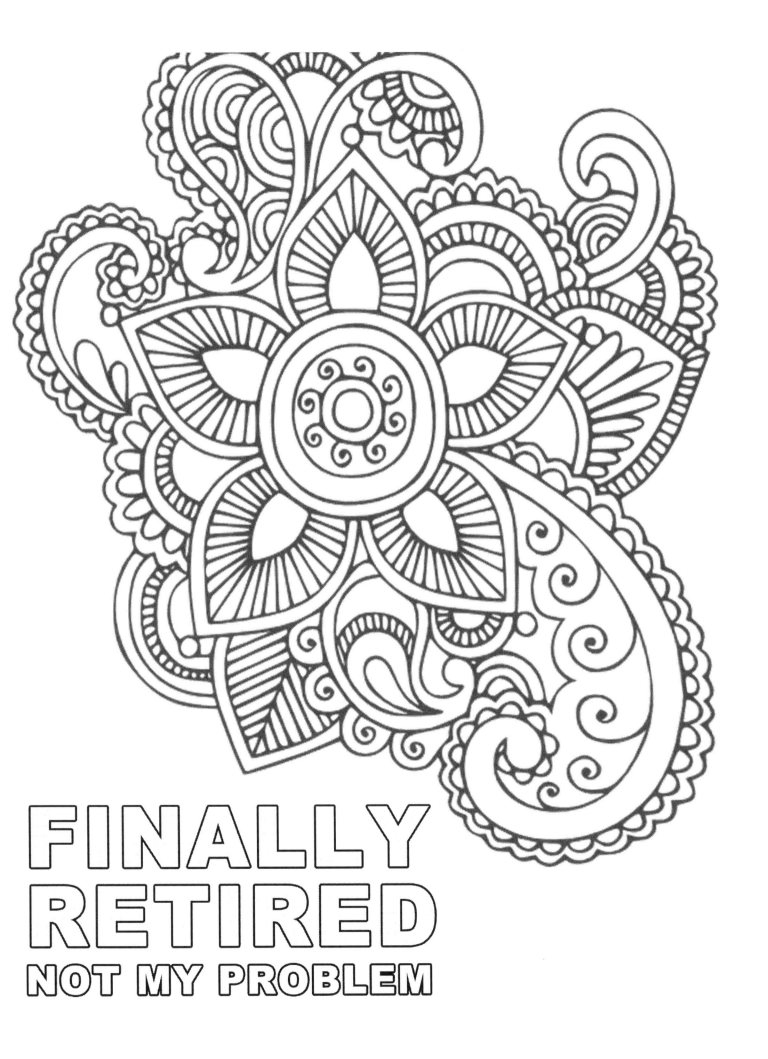

FINALLY
RETIRED
NOT MY PROBLEM

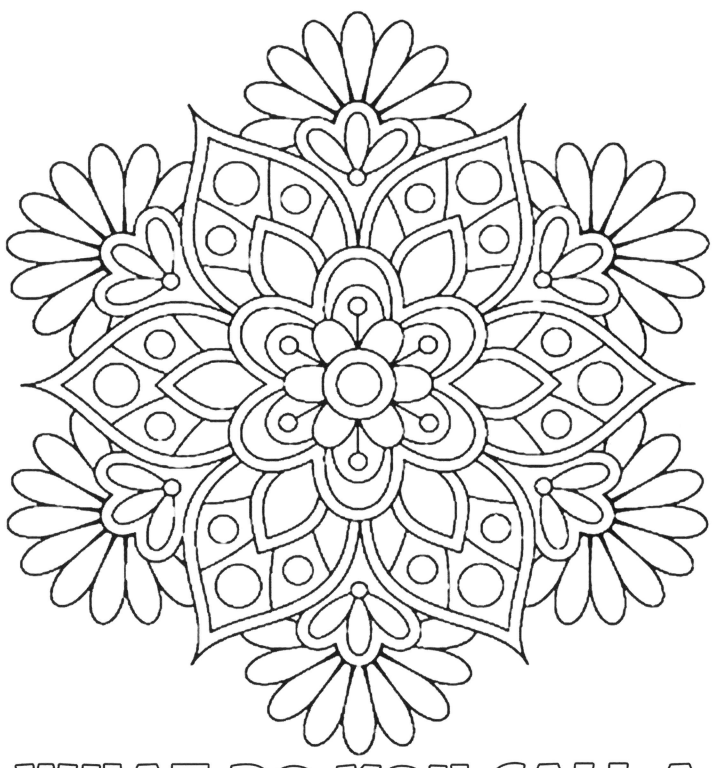

WHAT DO YOU CALL A PERSON WHO IS HAPPY ON MONDAY? RETIRED.

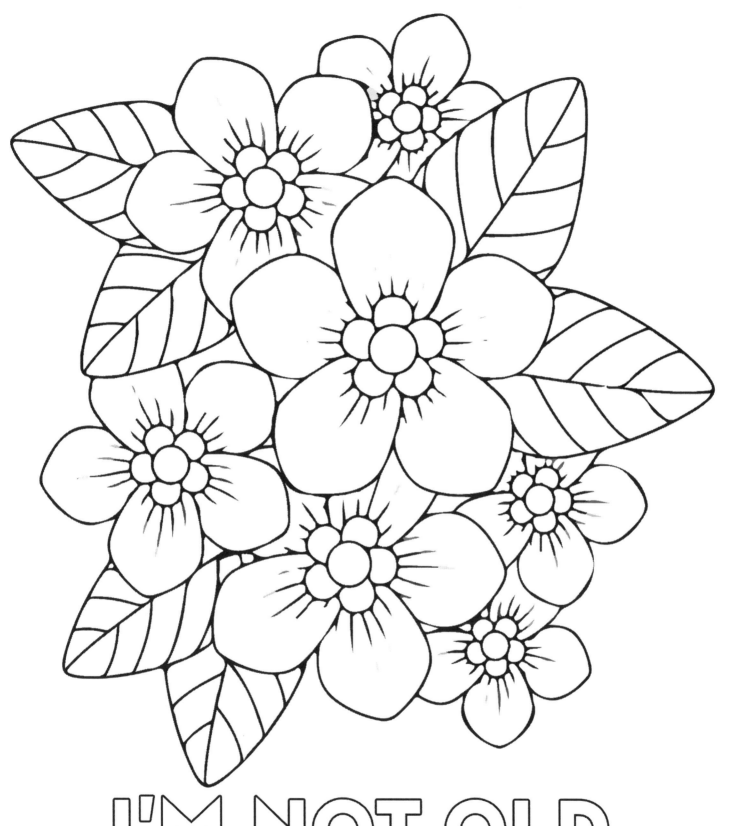

I'M NOT OLD
I'm a recycled teenager

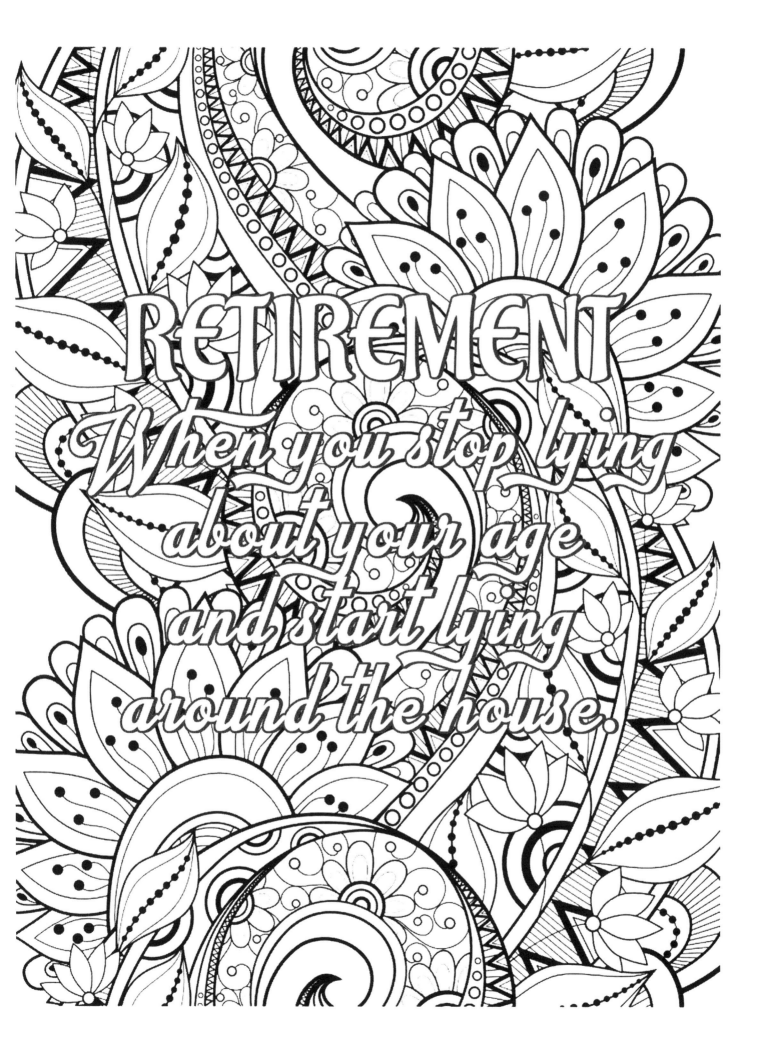

RETIREMENT
When you stop lying
about your age
and start lying
around the house.

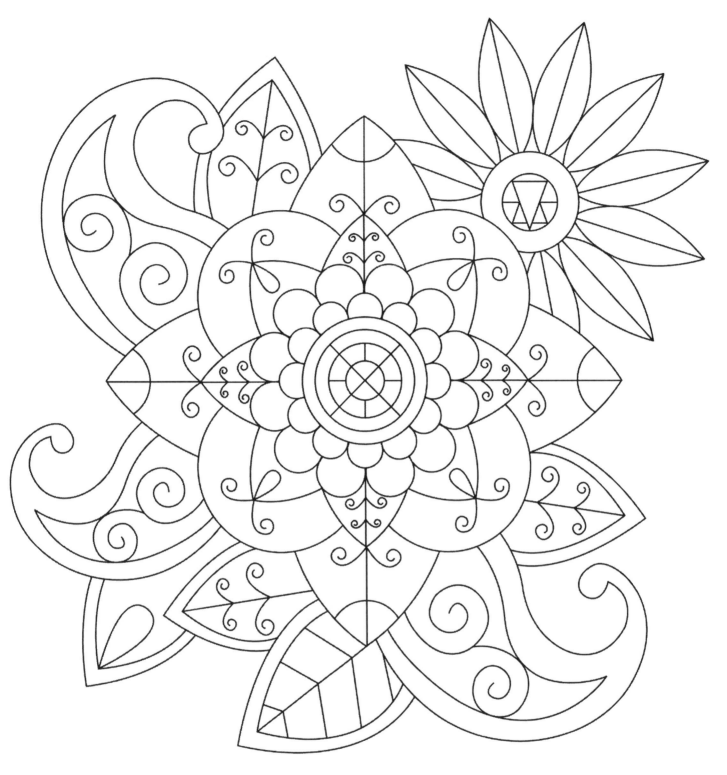

THE ONLY TROUBLE WITH RETIREMENT IS YOU NEVER GET A DAY OFF!

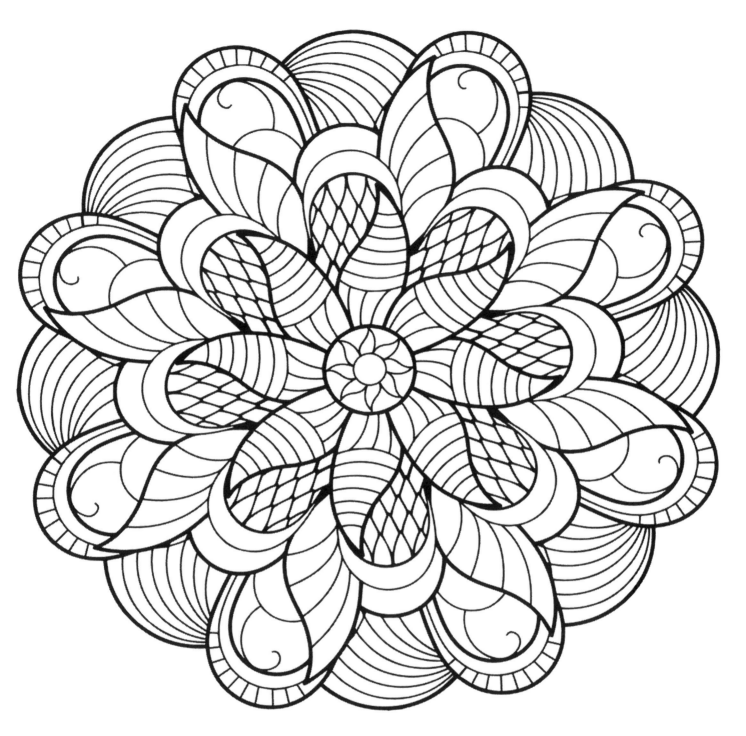

RETIREMENT
HALF THE MONEY
TWICE THE SPOUSE

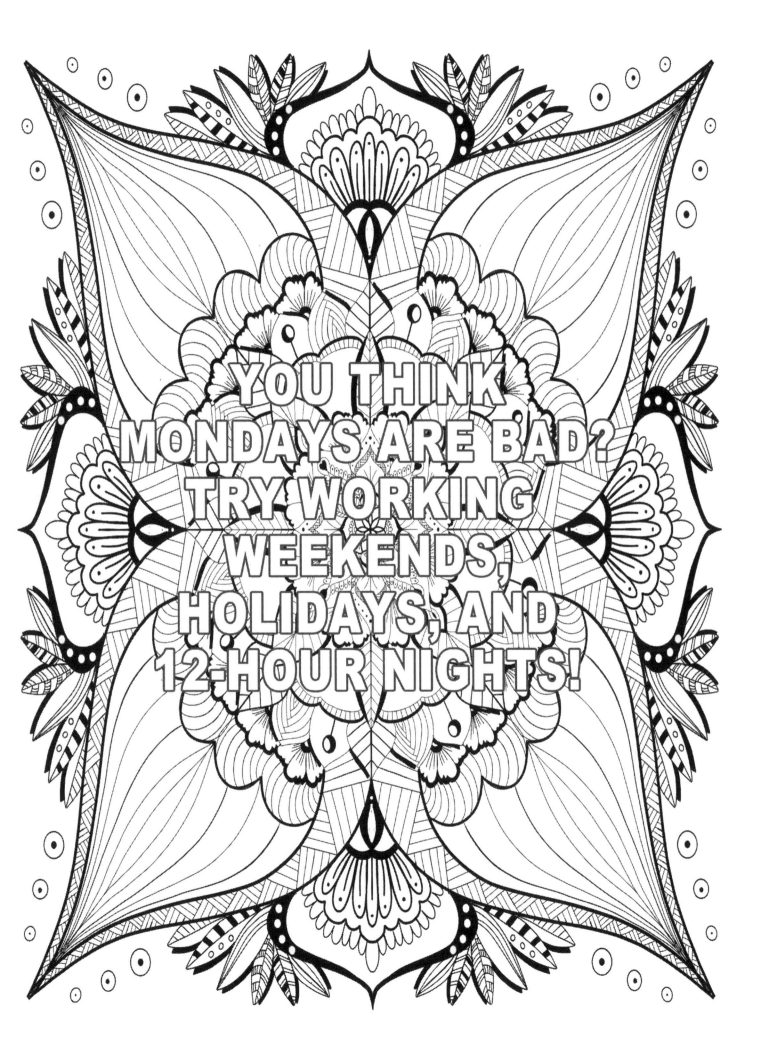

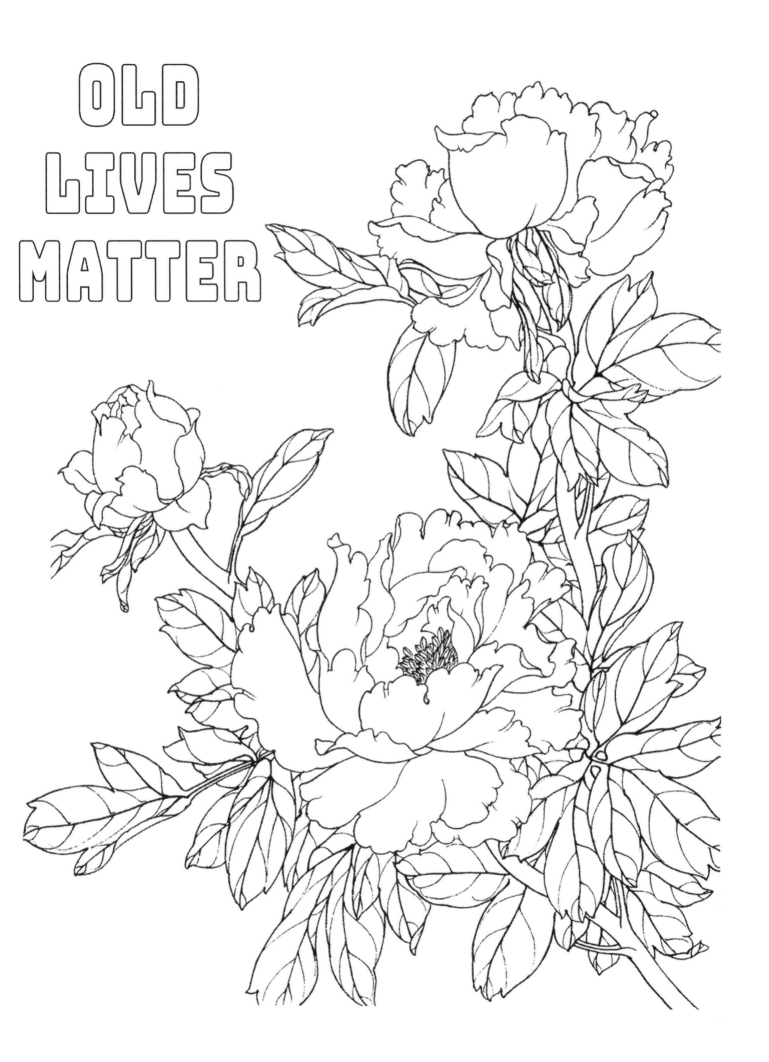

OLD
LIVES
MATTER

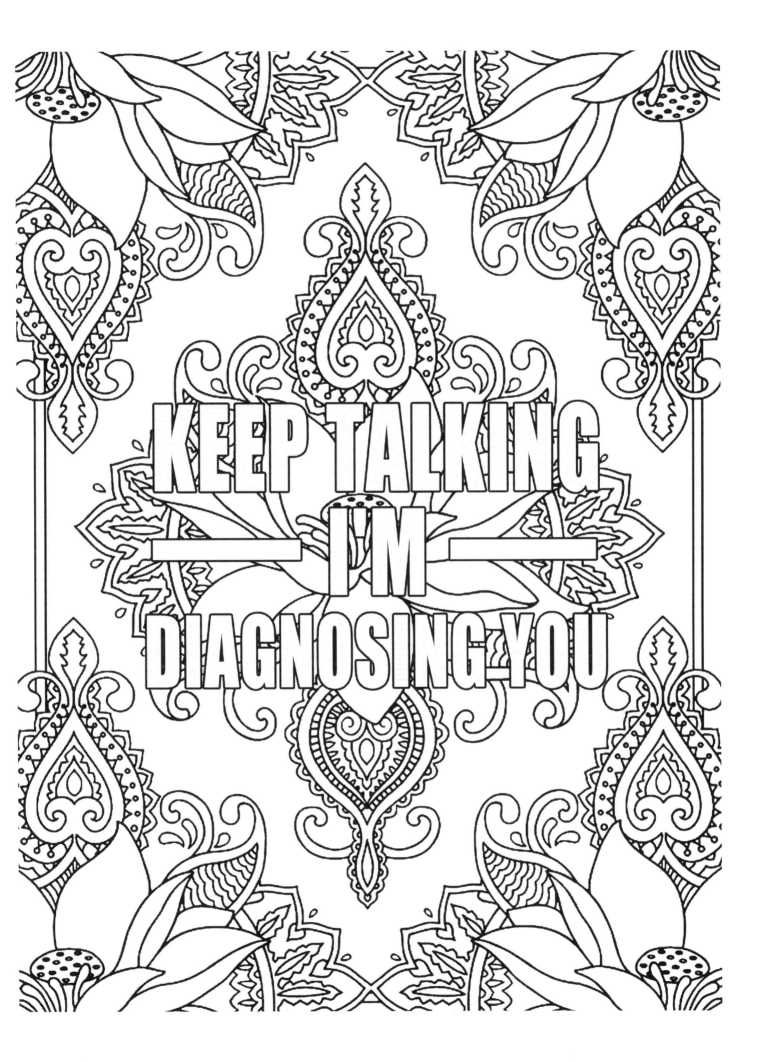

Made in United States
Orlando, FL
07 February 2022

14538047R00057